THE PANCAKE

A LOWER-BODY FLEXIBILITY STANDARD

Elia Bartolini

Copyright © 2023 by Elia Bartolini

All right reserved.

ISBN: 9798375902258

*"Do not go gentle into that good night,
Old age should burn and rave at close of day;
Rage, rage against the dying of the light.
Though wise men at their end know dark is right,
Because their words had forked no lightning they
Do not go gentle into that good night.
Rage, rage against the dying of the light."*

— Dylan Thomas

MORE FROM THE AUTHOR

DISCOVER ALL MY BOOKS!

Splits Hacking: the complete playbook to master the splits and your lower body flexibility.

Shoulders Range: the complete playbook to master your shoulders and upper body flexibility.

Balance your Handstand: the complete playbook to master your perfect freestanding handstand.

The V-sit: abs of steel and superhuman flexibility. Your complete guide toward the V-sit.

CONTENTS

MORE ABOUT THE AUTHOR — 1

HOW TO STRETCH & GAIN FLEXIBILITY — 3
Passive stretching — 6
PNF stretching — 8
Dynamic stretching — 12
Active stretching — 14
Loaded stretching — 19

THE PANCAKE STRETCH — 28
Lower body movements — 29
Anatomy of the pancake stretch — 30
Preparatory exercises — 36
Specific exercises — 72

WORKOUT TEMPLATES — 108
Beginner workout — 110
Intermediate workout — 113
Advanced workout — 116
How to organize your workouts — 119

ACKNOWLEDGMENTS — 125

MORE ABOUT THE AUTHOR

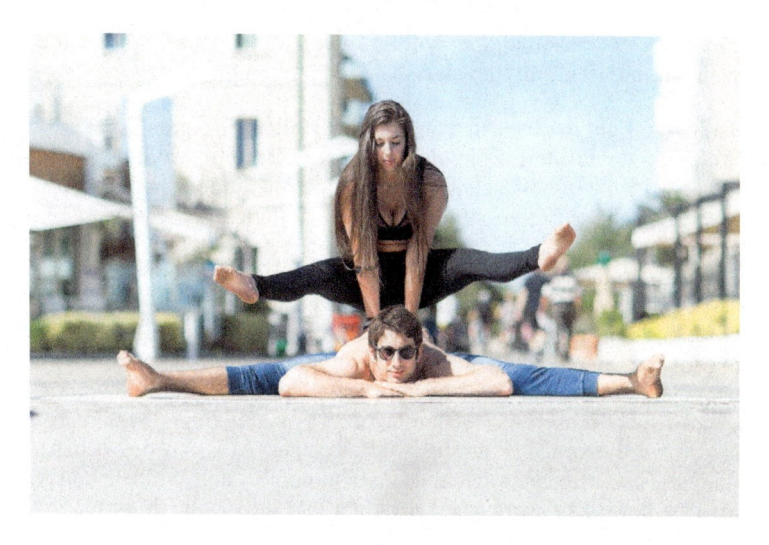

Figure 1. The Pancake Stretch.

Hey! Welcome to the pancake training guide: the complete guide where you'll learn how to correctly perform a pancake stretch. I'm Elia Bartolini, and I'm the author of this little guide.

The title of this book says it all "a lower-body flexibility standard" the pancake is one of the most important flexibility positions you can learn, and not by chance. There are so many positions the human body can do that take advantage of this type of flexibility, spread across a wide range of disciplines, from gymnastic to martial arts and many others.

It is a lower-body flexibility standard because it stretches a wide variety of muscles in your legs, hips and lower trunk, making your entire lower body super flexible.

It is my intention, throughout this book, to teach you how the pancake stretch works from an anatomical point of view, showing you the muscles involved and how your joints move during the pose. Then, to show you a path to follow to develop the flexibility you need in order to achieve the flat pancake stretch. Have a good read!

WHAT THIS BOOK IS ABOUT

This book is a roadmap that will bring you to the pancake, no matter your starting flexibility level. It is divided into 4 main parts.

The **first part** will teach you how to stretch and gain flexibility. We're going to start from the basics of flexibility training, what happens inside of a muscle when you stretch it, and then we're going to explore the different stretching methodologies you can use. Yes, you can stretch in many different ways! For instance, you can stay in a given stretching position and hold that stretching position, just staying there feeling the stretch for a given amount of seconds, basically doing nothing except stretching. That's passive stretching, one of the easiest stretching methodologies. But you can also use weights during your stretches, for example. You can voluntarily contract your muscles to relax more during a stretching position. You can move dynamically during your stretches. You can do so many things! These are the stretching methodologies, and we're going to explore how they work and why they can drastically improve our flexibility.

In the **second part**, we're going to analyze the pancake stretch from an anatomical point of view, understanding what the main muscles involved are and how your joints move during the stretching position.

In the **third part**, we're going to see the preparatory and specific exercises you can do to achieve the pancake stretch.

Finally, in the **fourth and last part**, I'm going to provide you with different workout ideas you can use to give your body a good stretch and achieve the pancake.

Sounds good? All right, let's go. Let's first understand how to stretch and what are the stretching methodologies.

PART 1 - HOW TO STRETCH

HOW TO STRETCH & GAIN FLEXIBILITY

I'm first sorry to those of you who don't like scientific literature. I really want to say that I don't like it too much either, as I'm more of a practical guy, but when it comes to the theory of stretching, I do think it's important to be a little more specific and call the various things with their respective names and nomenclatures.

Stretching is a common activity used by athletes, older adults, rehabilitation patients, and anyone participating in a fitness program. While the benefits of stretching are known, controversy remains about the best type of stretching for a particular goal or outcome, which is to say, what is the best **stretching methodology** to use.

Human movement is dependent on the amount of range of motion (ROM) available in your joints. In general, ROM may be limited by 2 anatomical entities: **joints** and **muscles**.

- **Joint restraints** include joint geometry and congruency, as well as the *capsuloligamentous* structures that surround the joint.

- **Muscle** provides both **passive and active tension**:

    - *Passive muscle tension* is dependent on the structural properties of the muscle, its surrounding fascia (more about that in a few lines) and the ligaments and tendons that connect the muscle to the bone.

    - *Active muscle tension* is provided by muscular contraction, both voluntary and involuntary.

Structurally, muscle has viscoelastic properties that provide passive tension. Think about it like an elastic band: it can lengthen, but up until a point, simply because it's made that way. Active tension instead results from the neuroreflexive properties of muscle, which is to say, the activation of the neurons that send signals to the brain to contract the muscles. These neurons can be fired both voluntarily (for instance, by deciding to contract a specific muscle) and involuntarily (for instance, when a great amount of muscular tension in a stretching position is recorded by the brain, it immediately sends signals in order to contract that specific muscle).

Muscle *"tightness"* results from an increase in tension from **active and/or passive mechanisms**. Passively, muscles can become shortened through postural adaptation or scarring; actively, muscles can become shorter due to spasms or contractions. Regardless of the cause, tightness limits the range of motion and may create a muscle imbalance.

Generally speaking, **stretching focuses on increasing the length of a muscle or muscles**, increasing the distance between a muscle's *origin* and *insertion* (more of which in each of this book's chapters regarding the anatomy of the positions). In terms of stretching, muscle tension is usually inversely related to length: the more you stretch a muscle, the greater the tension, and vice versa. Of course, when we talk about tension generated by the stretching effect, we're not talking only about muscles but also about other structures, such as the *joint capsule and fascia*, which are made up of different tissue than muscles with different biomechanical properties.

The *joint capsule* is what connects the muscle to the bone. That connection is made possible through a series of tendons and ligaments, which are structures made of connective tissue.

The *fascia*, instead, is a thin layer of connective tissue that surrounds our muscles. It prevents friction between the different muscle fibers and between the muscles themselves.

With that said, throughout this book, you're going to learn everything you have to know about **range of motion construction**: how to stretch your muscles and loosen up your joint restraints to create more flexibility. The first step we have to take is to understand the stretching methodologies and how they work.

STRETCHING METHODOLOGIES

In the previous chapter, I've explained what gaining flexibility means from a theoretical point of view. You have to understand now what to do in practice, though, which is something extremely more specific. As a matter of fact, you might understand the principles behind flexibility training, but if you want to make them happen, what should you do? How should you train? How long should you hold the stretching poses? How many times? How many workouts per week?

As you can see, there are many topics that deserve our attention at this point, and the stretching methodologies get really useful right now.

Stretching methodologies are the expression of theory into practice. They guide you during a flexibility workout, they tell you what to do, and they let you gain more range of motion.

We'll discover and study what, for me, are the best stretching methodologies out there, which you're also going to use throughout the various stretching positions explained and illustrated in this book.

PASSIVE STRETCHING

Passive stretching is the basis of all the other methodologies. It consists in staying in a given stretching position passively, without moving your body, trying to increase the range of motion gradually, breath after breath. During a passive stretching position, remember to breathe deeply, relax your muscles, don't tense 'em up, and try to find a new range of motion, going deeper into the stretch every 5/6 breaths.

INTENSITY AND STRETCHING

Even if relaxing is ok... You shouldn't sleep in a stretching position, though! Make sure the position itself is intense enough to challenge you and let you gain range of motion over time. In stretching, "intensity" refers to the amount of stretch and discomfort we feel in a given stretching position. On an intensity scale ranging from 1 to 10, we want a stretching position to sit between 6 and 9.

- Below 6, there's not a strong reason for your body to adapt to that stimulus because it isn't strong enough to induce an adaptation response.

- In the same manner, an intensity of 10 is too far beyond the adaptation curve, and your body can't adapt to a stimulus that is too far from your reach.

With that said, let me explain to you how to understand the intensity of a stretching position. I would say that there are 3 different kinds of intensity:

1. **Low intensity**, which means approximately 6/7 on our intensity scale.
   In a low-intensity stretching position, you should feel a gentle stretch in the muscles involved in the position, and you could spend a lot of time there. This range is good when you want to "normalize" a stretching position. By "normalize," I mean spending time in a given stretching position to adapt your CNS (Central Nervous System, which is your brain, responsible for your flexibility level) to that range and to feel less and less discomfort over time. Low-intensity stretching is really

important for long-term flexibility gains because, thanks to it, you will build your relaxed, "standard" range of motion. Even though it is important, it's not the best way to gain flexibility: oftentimes, you need more intensity to make a change and gain more flexibility.

2. **Medium intensity**: approximately 7/8 on our intensity scale.
   In a medium-intensity stretching position, you should feel a deep stretch sensation in the muscles involved in the position. You neither want to spend an eternity there nor want to exit after a few seconds. Make sure to relax the muscles involved in the stretch with nice and controlled breaths and a deep internal focus.
   The medium-intensity range is where most of your flexibility practice should stay. Here you have a really nice balance between intensity, CNS relaxation, and time spent in the position. A medium-intensity passive stretching position may be done between PNF or antagonist contractions, during a loaded stretching exercise, or after a dynamic stretch, just to mention some stretching methodologies we're going to discover in a few pages, so it's also good to when combined with different stretching techniques.

3. **High intensity**, which equals 9 on our intensity scale.
   A high-intensity stretching position should feel very uncomfortable. You should feel an intense stretch in the muscles involved in the position, and the amount of time you could spend in that position should be very low.
   The high-intensity range could be used, for example, in the final part of a PNF sequence, when right after the last PNF contraction, you keep the hardest stretching position you can achieve. Or it might be used to stay in a hard stretching position for some low-duration sets. Don't worry if you don't understand what I'm referring to with the words "PNF" or "Antagonist Contraction" yet because, again, we're going to discover their meaning in the next pages. This range of intensity, in my opinion, shouldn't be used a lot since it's really taxing on your body. With this range alone, you can't spend enough time in a stretching position to produce flexibility adaptations. Its best use is in combination with other techniques.

The secret to making passive stretching effective is understanding the intensity of a stretching position, ensuring that we're spending the right amount of time and effort in a certain stretching position to produce flexibility adaptations.

> **Remember**: we don't want to sleep in a stretching position. Make it hard, but not until the point you can't hold it. You should feel just a moderate discomfort. Putting it on a scale from 1 to 10, you should feel it between 6 and 8.

PNF STRETCHING

PNF stands for **Proprioceptive Neuromuscular Facilitation**, and it's one of the best ways to stretch and relax your body in a stretching position. It consists in voluntarily contracting the muscles involved in a stretching position for a given amount of time, usually expressed in seconds. The technical notes on how to do it and which muscles to contract will be covered specifically in each drill we're going to see, so don't bother about it since now it's important to understand how PNF works, how to do the muscle contractions and for how long.

First of all, you want to be in a stretching position to apply a **PNF contraction**. In that position, you want to contract the muscles you're stretching. The muscle contraction is isometric, which means that you hold it with a constant force being applied. A PNF contraction must be not maximal but medium and super specific for the muscles involved in the stretch. On a scale from 1 to 10, **keep it at 6/8**: start the contraction with an intensity of 6 and increase it after a few seconds. Reach the peak (8), hold it, and before you stop the contraction, slowly decrease its intensity.

The duration of a PNF contraction can vary from 10 to 20 seconds depending on the stretch and the muscles involved: the larger and stronger the muscle or muscles, the longer the contraction.

Every PNF contraction must have a relaxation phase before it (don't start a stretch immediately with a PNF). When it ends, relax, decrease the stretch a little bit, breath in, and on the breath out, get deeper into the stretch, reaching a new, more intense position. After this process, always start a new relaxation phase, which means that you passively stay in the stretch for a given amount of seconds or breaths. After that relaxation phase, you can start another PNF cycle or end the stretch there.

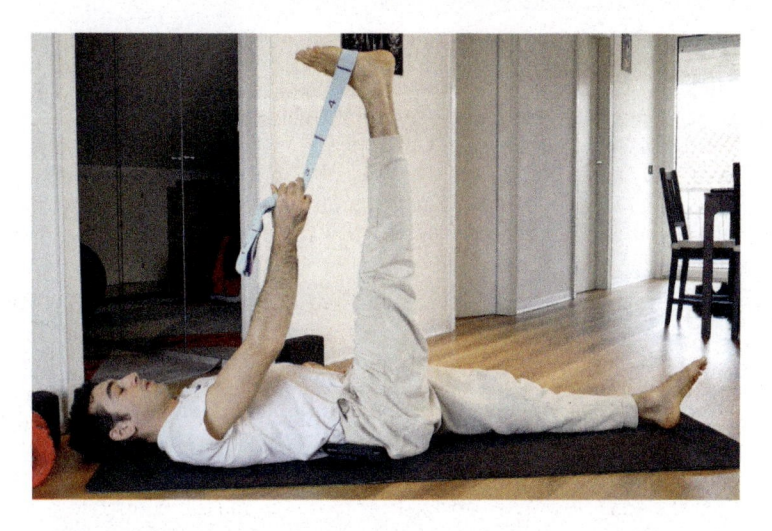

Figure 2. Example of PNF contraction during a stretching exercise.

QUICK EXAMPLE...

To give you a quick example, let's assume I want to apply a PNF contraction in the position of *figure 2*, where I'm stretching my hip extensors (hamstrings and glutes mostly), pulling my leg towards my body. To apply the PNF, I'll push the foot on top away from me, against the band's resistance, for a count of 10 to 20 seconds. I'll hold an isometric contraction starting with an intensity of 6 and slowly reaching 8.

Once the seconds are over, I'll stop the contraction, inhale, and on the exhale (it's really important you take just a moment to relax and almost immediately go into the stretch again!) I'll try to get deeper into the stretch, gaining some range of motion and relaxing in the position (passive stretch or relaxed phase).

After a PNF contraction, the inhale and/or exhale part should take no more than 2/4 seconds before going again in the stretching position. Right after the PNF contraction, the new stretching position must be passive and relaxed (**medium** intensity) for another 6 to 8 breaths. Then, you can start another PNF contraction or just end the PNF cycle there. The most important thing is to always finish with a passive phase and never with a PNF contraction.

A crucial aspect of a PNF contraction is the range of motion gained after the contraction itself: you should make a PNF contraction only if you can gain some range of motion right after it. If that's not the case, then there's no business in applying it, given that it also taxes your body and CNS. That's why I usually suggest doing from 1 to 3 PNF contractions at max in a given stretching position: if you do more, you're probably not going to gain any more range.

WHY DOES PNF WORK?

It's scientifically proven that performing a muscle contraction while the muscle is in an elongated position inhibits the protecting action of our CNS, which always holds some tension in a muscle or muscles during a stretching position to prevent possible damage.

As a matter of fact, muscles can be extended to about 130 percent of their resting length and can be contracted to about 70 percent of that same length.

The reason why a PNF contraction works is due to a phenomenon called **post-contractive reflex depression**. "Immediately after a sufficiently strong contraction, the muscle's resistance to elongation is momentarily reduced, and we can stretch further than would otherwise be the case." (Kit Laughlin, 2014). Immediately after a PNF contraction, a muscle can stretch slightly further thanks to the post-contractive reflex depression, a phenomenon that acts on the brain, the major responsible for flexibility gains and ranges of motion.

Let me put it more in simple terms. Imagine your CNS as a thoughtful person who always takes care of your muscles. Your muscles can be lengthened, and every time they do so, they may hurt themselves. So what does your CNS do? It monitors their length, and when that length reaches a certain point where potential damage might occur, the CNS contracts the muscles and stops their length there.

And here comes the magic. What if, instead of your CNS, you voluntarily contracted those muscles? Well, there wouldn't be any reason for the CNS to contract them anymore! As a matter of fact, a muscle contraction is already happening. So that thoughtful person who always takes care of your muscles' health would think, "these muscles are already contracting. There's no need for my intervention here!" And it would release a little bit of tension, allowing you to get deeper into a stretching position. The contraction you voluntarily do is called PNF, and now you know why it works: it tricks your brain a little bit, letting you gain more range of motion.

DYNAMIC STRETCHING

Dynamic stretching consists in moving your body between different positions to create a stretching effect in the muscles involved during that movement.

The process of entering and exiting in a stretching position is proved to be extremely beneficial for the relaxation of the muscles involved in the stretch and the release of the fascia, which is an extremely important component of the muscles.

You may wonder… Why the body relaxes more if we move our body parts during a stretching position? The answer is that sometimes a stretching position is particularly hard to maintain: if you stay there isometrically, without moving your body, the discomfort you feel from the hardness of the position might tense up the muscles involved in the stretch even more.

Vice versa, by entering and exiting from the positions, the muscles can rest a bit between them, and as a consequence, they can preserve a more relaxed state. Moreover, the fascia seems to relax better if little, gentle, and dynamic movements are provided during a stretching position.

There are two main types of dynamic stretching:

1. **Intermittent-Stretch** dynamic stretching.

2. **Continuous-Stretch** dynamic stretching.

The **Intermittent-Stretch** dynamic stretching consists in performing a movement that basically has two main positions: one where there's no stretch in the muscles on another where there's a stretch.
Let's take a squat as an example of this first type of dynamic stretching: as you may know, the squat has two main positions: the standing position, where there's no stretch, and the squat position, where there's a stretch. So, if you perform a squat motion, you'll feel the stretch only in the bottom part of the movement, not in the standing position, and that's how an intermitted stretch basically works.

In a **Continuous-Stretch** dynamic stretch, your body is constantly under stretch.

Take the cossack squat as an example, as shown in *figure 3*. When I start (1), I have my right leg bent and my left leg straight. Both legs are stretched, but each one is in a different way. As I change the position, going to the other side (3), the stretch changes, as now is the opposite of the starting position, but it's still present.

Since what we care about the most in this book is gaining flexibility, a particular focus should be put on the stretched position of a dynamic movement because that's where the flexibility gains happen.

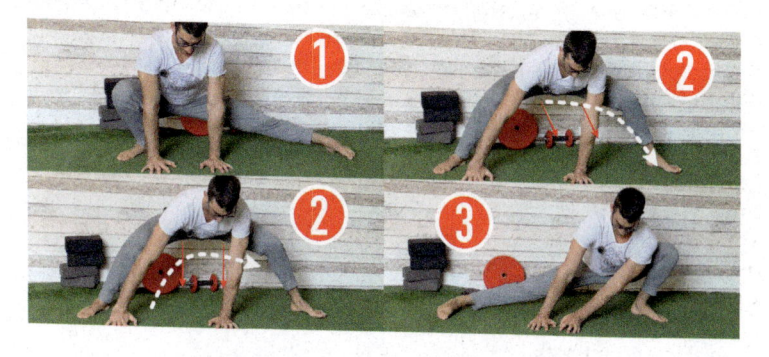

Figure 3. A cossack squat transition from right to left.

For this reason, you want to make sure to enter the stretched position with control and awareness of where you should feel the stretch, remain in the stretch for a bit (usually a couple of seconds), trying to stretch your muscles at your best, then exit from the position with control.

Now, take a closer look at the cossack squat. As you can see, as I do the transition (2), a unique stretch takes place in my hips as the result of the dynamic motion. Oftentimes, this is the biggest advantage of dynamic stretches: they allow you to explore stretches and positions that would be otherwise impossible to do and to reach with passive and/or static stretching exercises.

ACTIVE & ANTAGONIST STRETCHING

An active stretch is a stretch where a muscle contraction (**active contraction**) creates a stretch in another muscle (or muscles).

When it comes to active stretching, remember this little rule of thumb: most of the time, the muscles being stretched are the opposites of the ones being contracted, which are also called **"antagonist"** muscles.

I think that with a short example, you can better understand the idea of **Active Stretching**. Take at the two photos below: in the first one, I'm lifting one leg in front of me, and in the second one I straighten my knee. To do this movement, I need to contract my hip flexors (the muscles in the front part of my leg), and this creates a stretch in my hip extensors (hamstrings and glutes mostly, don't be afraid if you still don't know where are these muscles, we're going to discover it really soon), in the back part of my leg.

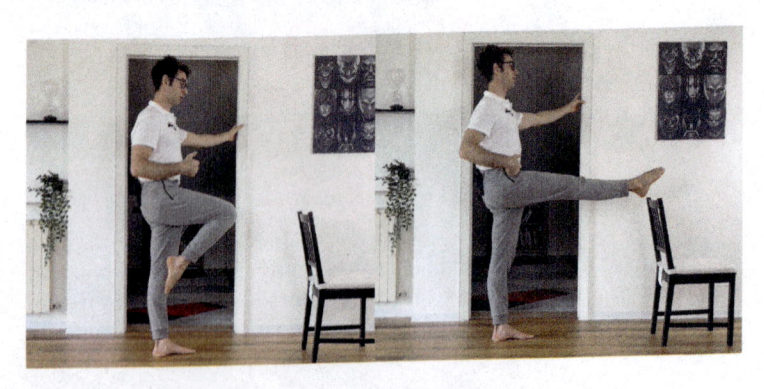

Figure 4. Active Hip Flexion.

I think there are 2 main ways of using an active muscle contraction to gain more flexibility.

1. In the above example, I create a stretch by moving one part of my body at its end range using an *active muscle contraction*. In this specific case, I'm using my hip flexors (*quads, iliopsoas, abs*) to lift my leg and, consequently to stretch my hip extensors. This is not a very strong stretching technique since

the only strength of the opposite muscles is, most of the time, not sufficiently strong to create a good stretch on the opposite ones. Hence, I wouldn't use it to build more flexibility. Still, I'd certainly use it to build strength in stretched positions, like holding active splits, an overhead squat, or to improve positions where active flexibility is needed.

Before I move on, though, I think it's important to clarify what I mean by "*active stretching positions*".

Take a look at the pictures down below. In order to perform these positions, the body requires a good level of **active flexibility**, which is the ability to maintain a given body part in a stretched position using the muscles' strength. As you can see from the pics down below, there's nothing that helps me go into the positions: I'm relying on my muscles' strength to get and stay there.

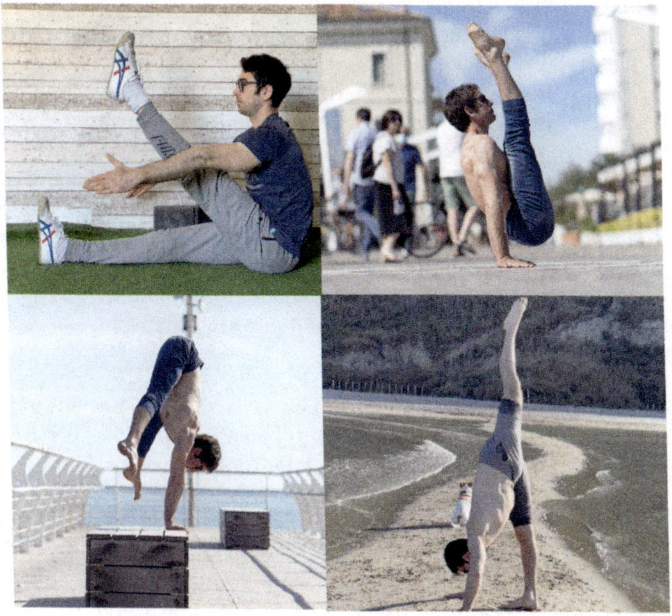

Figure 5. Different examples of active flexibility.

2. We can use an **active contraction** during a **stretching position** to gain more range of motion. This methodology is called "*Antagonist Stretching*". Let's see how it works. First of all, there are scientifically-proven studies that show how contracting the antagonist muscles of the ones involved in a stretching position produces a relaxing effect on the muscles you're stretching, allowing you to relax more and get deeper into a stretching position.

This, of course, implies that you have to be in a stretched position if you want to successfully apply this methodology, and once there, you have to contract the opposite muscles of the ones being stretched to obtain a relaxation effect. So far, so good, right? But there's more. As a matter of fact, using the *antagonist stretching* methodologies carries two main benefits.

The first benefit is the **relaxation effect** (which we've talked about so far), thanks to which you can gain more range of motion thanks to the antagonist contraction.

The second benefit is the **strength-construction effect**. Contracting the antagonist muscles at the end range of a certain joint or movement (which means the max range of motion a certain joint can express) will strengthen your muscles and improve the control you have over that range of motion. Better control and strength in a given position equal better chances to gain flexibility and keep the joints healthy and strong in the long term.

Now, let's talk about how the **Antagonist Contraction (AC)** should be done. Actually, there are two main ways to use an antagonist contraction:

1) The first one is much similar to a PNF. The antagonist contraction is held **isometrically**, and, as for the PNF, you should ramp up the intensity of the contraction as it goes on: start from an intensity of 6/7 and reach 9 (on a scale from 1 to 10). Keep it slightly harder compared to a PNF contraction. Hold the contraction for 10 to 20 seconds, then release it and continue the stretch passively without squeezing the muscles anymore. Repeat the process 2 to 5 times, much like in a PNF, trying to gain some range of motion after every antagonist contraction.

2) Keep a gentle and **continuous antagonist contraction** for the whole duration of the stretch. Especially when it comes to advanced stretching positions, keeping a gentle antagonist contraction does help to control the position, decrease pain and discomfort, and relax the muscles involved in the stretch.
In this case, I suggest holding a low-intensity (2 to 5 on our intensity scale) contraction for 30 seconds to 1 minute.
You can use this principle in every stretching position you know: when you are in a given stretching position, squeeze your antagonist muscles gently, and you're surely going to feel the difference: the muscles you're trying to stretch will "magically" relax more.

The applications of active stretching vary according to each practitioner's purpose: the most important thing is understanding the difference between an active stretch and an active contraction.

An active stretch is a stretching position where a muscle contraction **creates** the stretch, and there are several active stretches out there. We're going to see some examples throughout the book, and I hope the concept will get clearer and clearer.

An active contraction, more specifically an antagonist contraction, instead, is something you can do during a stretching position to better relax your muscles and gain more range of motion.

PASSIVE VS ACTIVE FLEXIBILITY

At this point, I do think it's essential to understand that active flexibility is **directly correlated** with passive flexibility. Again, to clarify the concept I must say that with active flexibility, I mean the ability to move your body through a certain range of motion (imagine moving your legs at their maximal range of motion without using any kind of assistance).

Passive flexibility greatly influences active flexibility, and let me tell you why: in an active stretch, some muscles contract (*antagonists* of the stretch) to move a certain body part and create a stretch in the opposite muscles (agonists of the stretch) and if the muscles that oppose to this movement are stiff, the antagonists will have a rough time to move that body part: the more the muscles that are being stretched pull, the less you can move your body in a particular direction. That should be pretty logical, right? Vice versa, if the antagonists contract and the agonists are **soft and flexible**, the former will move the body easily and smoothly since they'll encounter less and less resistance coming from the latter.

Here's your take-home message: before you start thinking about *active flexibility*, make sure you have nice passive flexibility. Then, it will be much easier to gain active flexibility.

Many leg or hip-related movements require active leg or hip flexibility. The pancake demands a good level of hips and legs active flexibility, as well as many other exercises require active flexibility to be performed. That's why this chapter is very important to understand the logic behind some exercises we're going to explore throughout the book and to realize why some stretches are performed in such a way.

Now, let's move on. Let's understand how to stretch using weights and other kinds of assistance.

LOADED STRETCHING

Loaded stretching, in terms of execution, is almost identical to passive or dynamic stretching: you have to remain in a stretching position and try to get deeper and deeper into the stretch or move through different positions to gain range of motion, with the "only" huge difference that during a loaded stretching exercise a weight, the force of gravity, a partner, or your self-assistance may help you gain more range of motion.

The reason why loaded stretching helps you gain more flexibility is that it aims to let you find a sensation of stretch that, without an assistance, would have been impossible to reach. Think about it for a moment: have you ever felt like you couldn't get any further into a stretch, but as soon as someone pushed you down or you used a weight, all of a sudden, you could express more flexibility? Has it ever happened to you? Well, this is the principle behind loaded stretching.

First of all, I'd like to explain to you the concept of **loaded stretching** using as an example a stretch done with the assistance of a weight, as I think it's going to be much easier to understand and teach this way, but please take into consideration that loaded stretching can be performed with other kinds of assistance in addition to the weight.

Let's say that during a loaded stretching position, you want to use a weight to gain more range of motion. The amount of weight you may use is *critical*: make sure not to pick up a weight that is too heavy for you. If you choose a weight that is too heavy, you're probably going to resist the stretch and contract your muscles rather than letting your body relax and find a deep sensation of stretch. On the contrary, if you use a weight that is too light for you, there will be no real differences between a loaded stretching and a passive stretching position without a weight. Hence, there would be no business in using a weight, cause the intensity of the stretch would be the same as by not using it. The same is true for any kind of assistance you may use during a loaded stretch: make sure you feel it and that it helps you get deeper into the stretch.

Loaded stretching is a stretching technique that can be used alone or in combination with other stretching methodologies. For example, you can use a weight to find a deeper position in a given stretching position; then, once there, you can use some PNF contractions to gain range of motion. That's an example of combined loaded + PNF stretching. Many other variations are possible as well, like loaded + passive, loaded + dynamic, etc. We'll be talking about these combinations in great detail throughout the book as soon as they present themselves. All the other details, like how long to hold a position or how to move the body to find the correct sensation of stretch, will be covered specifically in each exercise's explanation.

WHY DOES LOADED STRETCHING WORK?

There are two ways you can use a weight to improve your flexibility in a given stretching position, but first of all, let me remind you what I said about the PNF to explain to you why it works: "Immediately after a sufficiently strong contraction, the muscle's resistance to elongation is momentarily reduced, and we can stretch further than would otherwise be the case. This phenomenon is called **postcontractive reflex depression** (PRD)."

With loaded stretching, we can create two very different stretches according to how we use the weight in the position. As a matter of fact, you can:

1) Let the weight **assist the position while you stay in a relaxed, passive stretch**. In this case, the PRD doesn't influence the stretch since there's no muscle contraction: you're trying to get relaxed and deeper into the stretch. This is a very effective way to stretch in combination with the passive stretching methodology. As a matter of fact, most of the time, the only force of gravity isn't sufficiently strong to create a good stretch on a certain body part: the assistance of a weight or another kind of external resistance does help quite a lot in this case, allowing you to get deeper into the stretch. Try to figure out this in your mind: you're lying down on your back on the floor with your legs against a wall in front of you, and you have some ankle weights wrapped around your ankles. The weights are pulling your legs down, opening them like in a split, right? Well, here you're using a weight to create a stretch (hence is passive stretching), and if you just stay passively there, trying to

increase your range of motion, you're using this first strategy.

2) **Create muscle tension**, both dynamically or isometrically, thanks to the weight's assistance or another kind of external force. In this case, the muscles do contract while they are in a stretching position, and so the PRD does influence the stretch, allowing your muscles to relax right after that contraction. Now, I know it might sound a little strange, so please let me clarify this second case with some examples to better understand what I'm talking about.

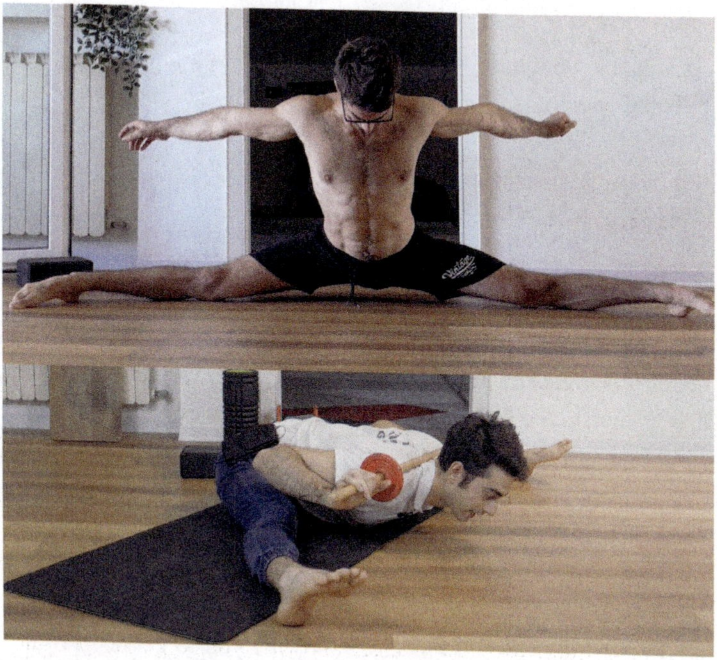

Figure 6. Two examples of loaded stretches.

Try to think about a side split where your legs don't touch the floor, and you hold the position with the only strength of them. In that case, you are in a stretching position, but your muscles are not relaxed or passive. On the contrary, they are working so hard to generate tension to hold your body in that position! This kind of muscle contraction is similar yet a little bit different from a PNF contraction.

It's similar because it's a muscle contraction that happens when the muscles are in an elongated state, and it's different because this is not a "fake" contraction: you don't voluntarily contract the muscle against some kind of imaginary resistance, as you do in a PNF, here you're contracting your muscles 'cause they have to if you want to keep holding that position!

You can see a clear example of a loaded stretching exercise where a real muscle contraction is going on in *figure 6*.

As you can see, I have to squeeze my legs' muscles to hold my body in that position. I'm not voluntarily contracting them (as in a PNF). I'm forced to do so!

But wait! I'm not using a weight in that position! Is it still considered a loaded stretching position? For sure! The load, in this case, is the product of gravity plus the leverage of my legs. Loaded stretching doesn't only stand for weighted stretching, as I said at the beginning of this chapter.

Now, take a look at the second picture in *figure 6*. My goal here is to hold the deepest stretch I can with the weight's pressure on my body: in this way, I have to contract my legs' muscles to remain in the stretch since, as you can see, I'm not touching the floor with my trunk. That muscle contraction will produce a lengthening effect immediately after it (as a result of the PRD), letting me gain some range of motion and/or comfort in the subsequent position as long as I put my trunk on the floor or some supports, letting it relax in the position.

We now know that a loaded stretching exercise could be done to **relax** the body and/or to **create muscle tension** in a stretched position. Both techniques generally work fine. They're just different, and we're going to use them both throughout this book.

PNF OR LOADED STRETCHING? WHICH ONE IS BETTER?

After hearing me saying that a loaded stretching position might be really similar to a PNF contraction, people often get confused. They ask me:" What should I do? A PNF contraction or a loaded stretching exercise? You've said that a PNF contraction is fake... I'm not gonna do it anymore!". Well, actually, I think that both are excellent techniques and each one of them has its own benefits. Let me clarify this a little bit better.

A PNF contraction is extremely specific, safe, and easy to do. Everyone can do it: beginners, intermediate, or advanced practitioners, and all of them can get really good results from it. It's specific because you can contract your muscles during a max or near-max range position, which means that you can create tension exactly at the *muscle length* you want and need to. This cannot happen in a loaded stretching position, where you can **create tension** only where you're strong enough to hold the position.

For these reasons, I would say that PNF is generally speaking more versatile and may be applied in many contexts and situations. Loaded stretching has many different applications as well. Remember that you can use it in two main ways: 1) to help you get deeper into a stretch and 2) to build strength and control in a stretched position. If you use the first option (to get deeper into a stretch), you can apply it to various stretching positions as you might be using a weight, a partner's assistance, or your own body to increase the intensity of the stretch.

To further explain the first application of loaded stretching, I'd like to provide you with an example that I always show people to let them understand how a stretch may be performed with the same technique but with different intentions. Take a look at the three pics you can see in *figure 7*. As you can see, these are all the same stretching positions.

In the first one, I'm in the stretch without any kind of assistance. In the second and third, I'm using an assistance to get deeper into the stretch, folding my trunk further towards my legs: my hands in the second pic, and a weight in the third one.

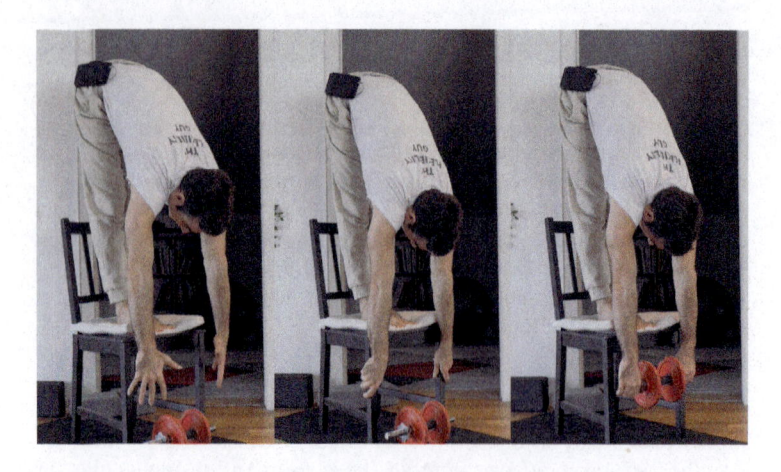

Figure 7. Same stretching position, 3 different ways to get into the stretch: no assistance, pulling with the hands, using a weight.

As you can see, the applications of loaded stretching are multiple.

LOADED STRETCHING AND WEIGHTS

Something you should remember when it comes to loaded stretching is that the purpose of a certain exercise may vary according to the weight you're using. As a matter of fact, there are roughly two main categories of weights you can use in a stretching position:

- **Light to Medium**: if you use a light to medium weight, that weight will help you stretch there without demanding tension from your muscles. These are the weights you should use if you want to *relax* in the stretch and get deeper.

- **Medium to Heavy**: Vice versa, if you use a medium-high weight, it will demand more tension coming from your muscles. As you'll go into the stretch, you'll feel that you have to control the weight in order to stay there. These are the weights you should use if you want to build flexibility and strength in the stretching position.

Can you see how the **amount of weight** you use impacts the final outcome of a stretch? The same exercise, done with a different weight, produces two different stretches and should be treated in a different way.

During your training, you can mix the two strategies of loaded stretching to obtain the best in terms of flexibility gains, and we're going to talk about it during the workout design section.

By the way, always remember that everything starts from the purpose of a stretch. If, throughout the book, I'll tell you, "your purpose is to relax during this position", you'll know that the amount of weight you should be using will be light to medium. Vice versa, if I'll tell you, "squeeze your muscles and stay in the position", then the suggested amount of weight is medium to heavy.

FIRST COMES THE "HOW" AND THEN THE "WHAT"

Here we are at the end of this long introductory chapter about stretching methodologies. Stretching methodologies are the basis of a flexibility practice: without them, you are lost in a world where you probably don't know what you're doing.

The first things people usually ask for a stretching position are: "How long should I stay there?" Or "What should I do here?".

Now, after this chapter, I hope you'll see a stretching position with completely different eyes. I hope you'll be able to understand that a stretching position itself means nothing if you don't know what to do there, like how intense it should feel and how you should apply a stretching methodology there.

Remember that first comes the "how," and then comes the "what." Try to understand how you should feel and apply a stretching methodology first, then think about the "what," that is, whatever stretching position you might be doing.

The magic happens in the "how," not in the "what." People think some magic exercises will change their life. Given that some exercises are better than others and you should select what you're doing carefully to achieve better results, the major difference is how you do your stuff; how you feel the stretch; how you apply your PNF contractions; how you use the weight during a loaded stretch; or how hard you go into the stretch when you have to. That makes the real difference, among many other things that we're going to discover more specifically throughout this book.

With that being said, we now have everything we need to understand better how to practice the stretching positions we're going to see next. Are you ready? Let's go.

> **Remember**: even the more basic exercises can still very useful for advanced trainees who want to improve their flexibility level.

MEASURE YOUR OWN PROGRESS

Something must be said about how to proceed through the exercises exposed in this book and how to deal with your progress. There's not a fixed, immutable rule that will tell you when to progress to another exercise or not: flexibility doesn't work this way. Even the more basic exercises might still be useful for advanced trainees who want to improve their flexibility level.

If you are a beginner, start with the first exercises you find in the book. Spend some time there, feel that your range of motion improves, and from time to time, like 6 to 8 weeks, give some harder positions a go. If you feel ok with them and you can keep a good technique (be honest with yourself, I will provide all the technical information for each and every exercise, but I can't be there with you. The most important thing is that you always make sure to practice with a good technique, and when you feel ready and comfortable in a stretch, change that stretch with a harder one and continue with your training. Don't try new stuff for another 6/8 weeks, then make a new test again. If things got better, perfect, change some easy exercises with harder ones and repeat. If things are still the same, don't worry. Give yourself more time, and keep following your workouts. Push a little bit harder in your stretches. Make sure you're not missing some technical points and that you're feeling a deep sensation of stretch during the exercises you're doing. Probably, you'll get results in several months, so don't be fooled by the hunger to constantly add new exercises: stick to some of them and build super flexibility there. When you feel confident with a harder variation, test it and move on.

The point here is that no magical exercise exists: you can stick to 3 exercises, done correctly with progression in the range of motion over time, and still reach your goals. Despite that, this is not a suggested path to follow since changing exercises gives your body a much wider variety of stimuli and reasons to progress, plus it adds fun and variety to the mix, which are fundamental things in everyone's training and life. Anyhow, this is pure theory. We don't want to be only theoreticians, guys. We're, first of all, practitioners. Make sure to put theory into work. That's why theory exists in stretching: to help us understand why and how to stretch and to make more flexibility gains, not for the only sake of more theory. Theory won't train flexibility for you, after all! Am I right?

Part 2

—

THE PANCAKE

LOWER BODY MOVEMENTS

In this book, you're going to find different terms: *hip flexion, hip extension, knee flexion, and hip abduction*, just to mention some. Here you can find a clear illustration of their meaning and almost all the lower-body movements you can do.

Come back here whenever you want to check and study these movements for visual reference.

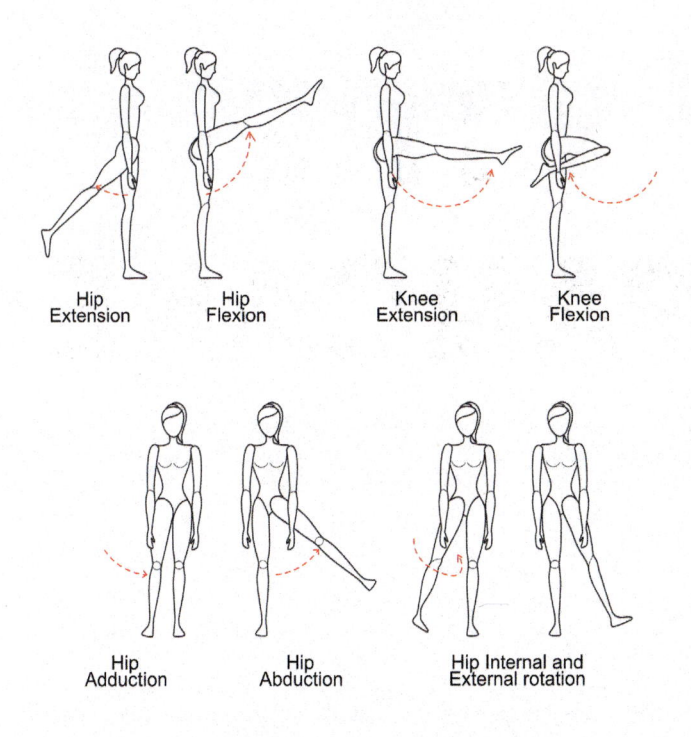

Figure 8. Lower-body movements.

Guys, how much I love these illustrations!

ANATOMY OF THE PANCAKE STRETCH

From an anatomical point of view, the pancake is the combination of two movements: *hip flexion*, and *hip abduction*. See *figure 8* for visual reference.

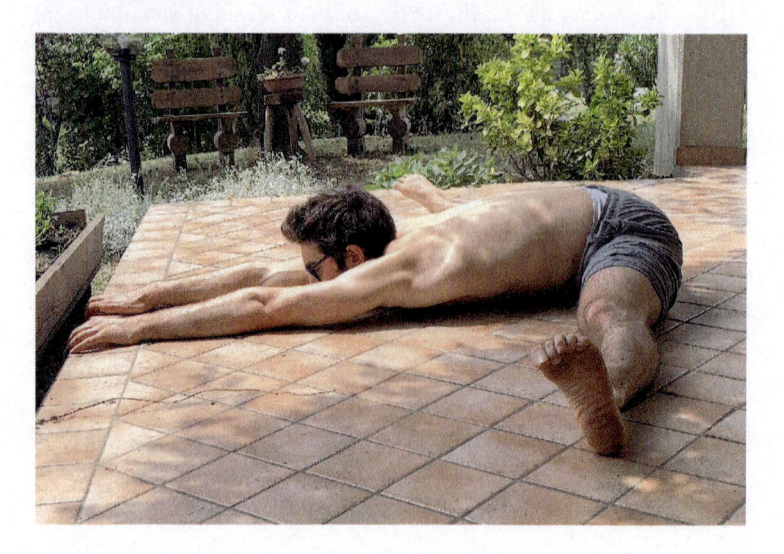

Figure 9. A flat pancake stretch.

As you can clearly see in *figure 9*, there are two movements happening at the same time: I'm flexing my trunk toward my legs, and this is hip flexion, while I'm spreading my legs wide apart, and this is hip abduction.

Now, a really important question we need to answer is: what are the major **muscles that oppose** to hip flexion and hip abduction? Knowing that, we can figure out what to work on to maximize the range of motion in the pancake stretch, right?

For **hip flexion**, the major muscles that oppose this movement are the *hamstrings* (*biceps femoris, semitendinosus, semimembranosus*) and the *glutes*, among many others, smaller muscles like the *piriformis*.

For **hip abduction**, the major muscles that oppose this movement are the *adductors* (*adductor magnus, adductor longus, adductor brevis, gracilis, pectineus*).

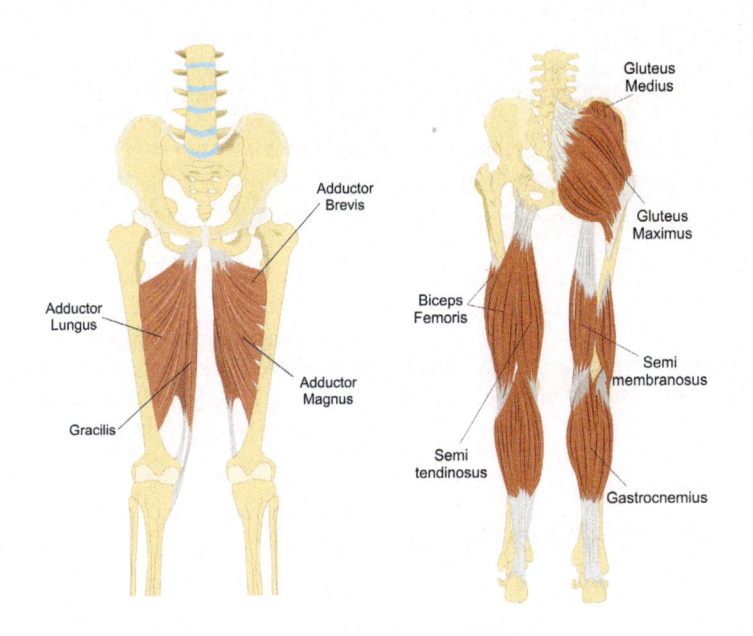

Figure 10. Anatomy of the adductors (left) and hip extensors (right).

We now know each and every muscle involved in this beautiful stretching position, and we can then focus on the development of the flexibility of these muscles taken both separately and as a whole. For example, if you're feeling that you can easily fold your trunk toward your legs, but your legs seem to have a bad time spreading wide apart, you know that the problem might be hip abduction and that the major muscles that limit that particular movement are the adductors, mostly. You can then focus on the exercises that specifically build adductors and legs-apart flexibility as a strategy to improve your pancake. Same reasoning for whichever movement you may feel stiffer and/or underdeveloped compared to the rest.

Once the flexibility of all the muscles involved in the position is sufficient, it's going to be tremendously easier for you to focus on the specific pancake exercises you have to do to reach the final position rather than trying them right from the start without having built a sufficient general flexibility level in the muscles involved in the pancake first.

> **Remember**: building at first a good general flexibility level in the muscles involved in a pancake stretch is important if you want to be successful with the specific exercises later on.

Even though in a pancake the major movements that interest us are hip flexion and hip abduction, we also have to consider that in a correct pancake, the legs must stay **completely straight**, which means extending the knees completely. As a consequence of that, also the **calves muscles** (*gastrocnemius in this case*) have to be flexible in order to maximize knee extension and prevent stiffness there.

PANCAKE TECHNIQUE

Let's talk about one of the most important things you have to know about the pancake stretch: the **positioning of your hips**. During a pancake, your hips must stay in an **anterior pelvic tilt**.

It is critical now that you understand the difference between a posterior and anterior pelvic tilt. Without getting too deep into the anatomical stuff, take a look at the two pictures in *figure 11*. Can you see how I'm sitting in different postures?

In a **posterior pelvic tilt**, I'm sitting down on my glutes, my lower back is rounded, and my abdominals are shortened.

In an **anterior pelvic tilt**, I'm sitting on top of my hip bones, my glutes are pushed back, my lower back is straight and slightly arched, and my abdominals are elongated.

This is how your hips must stay during a pancake position, something far from being easy, but that guarantees you a good amount of stretch in all the muscles involved in the position.

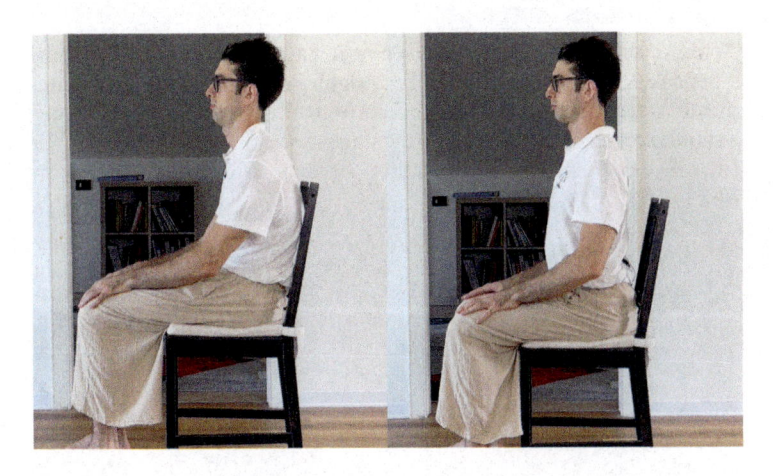

Figure 11. Posterior pelvic tilt (left) and anterior pelvic tilt (right) during a seated position.

Even though things may seem easy in theory, they're not in practice, as this type of activation is the result of two very important things.

1) **Flexibility**. Keeping an anterior pelvic tilt demands a good amount of flexibility both in your *hip extensors* (*hamstrings* and *glutes*) and *adductors*, along with other small muscles like the *piriformis*. That's why the pancake is so difficult! It's not only about flexing the body forward or spreading the legs apart, it's also about your pelvic rotation: you cannot achieve a flat pancake stretch if you don't move your hips into anterior pelvic tilt! And to anterior pelvic tilt, especially during a pancake stretch, you need high levels of flexibility.

2) **Muscles activation**: besides the flexibility requirements, you also need to understand and figure out how to move your body correctly and **activate your muscles** to obtain such a posture. Beware, though, that this muscle activation is a byproduct of your flexibility. Only with the right amount of flexibility can you figure out your hips' movements and how to control them. So, it is critical that you develop point number one first and simultaneously try to move your hips into the correct activation and see how it goes. That's why I make such a remarkable distinction between preparatory and specific exercises: with the preparatory, you develop the flexibility you need to figure out how to move correctly during the specific.

At this point, we know all that we need to know in order to develop a pancake: **hip flexion** flexibility (stretch your hamstrings and glutes mostly), **hip abduction** flexibility (stretch your adductors), **knee extension** (stretch your hamstrings and calves) and **anterior pelvic tilt** development (a combination of hamstrings and adductors flexibility).

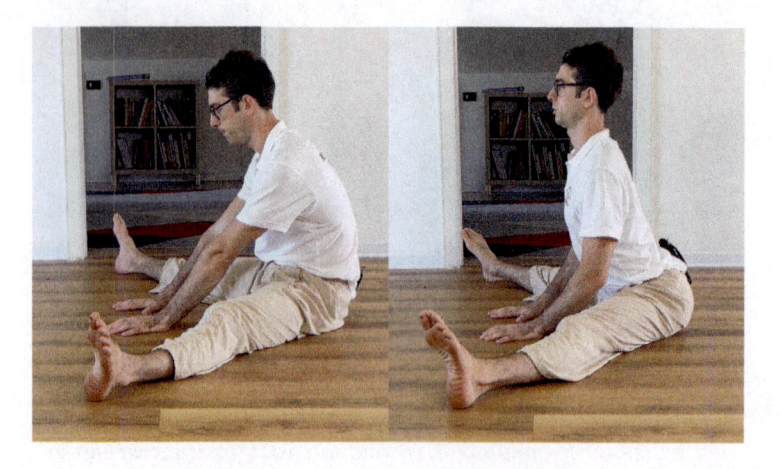

Figure 12. Posterior pelvic tilt (left) and anterior pelvic tilt (right) during a pancake position. Can you tell which one is the correct one?

Time to figure out now what are the best exercises you can do for your pancake stretch, starting with the preparatory ones and then getting deep into the specific ones. Ready? Go!

Part 3

—

PREPARATORY EXERCISES

HORSE STANCE

Start standing with your legs wide apart and your feet pointing slightly out. How much to widen your legs depends on your flexibility level: as a general rule of thumb, keep a wide stance, approximately 2 times your shoulders width to start with. From there, squat down, keeping your torso as upright as possible and driving both of your knees constantly out. Lower down your hips until they are in line with your knees, as you can see in the pictures on this page.

The most important thing about this hip mobilization exercise is **driving the knees out** at all times: squeeze the glutes muscles in order to do so, and don't let the knees go inwards. Once in the bottom position, you can use many different strategies to gain more range of motion and stretch the muscles involved in the position.

▸ **Put your hands on your knees** and push them out strongly. Relax the adductors muscles and let your legs spread wide apart: imagine opening them as if you wanted to reach a 180 degrees angle.

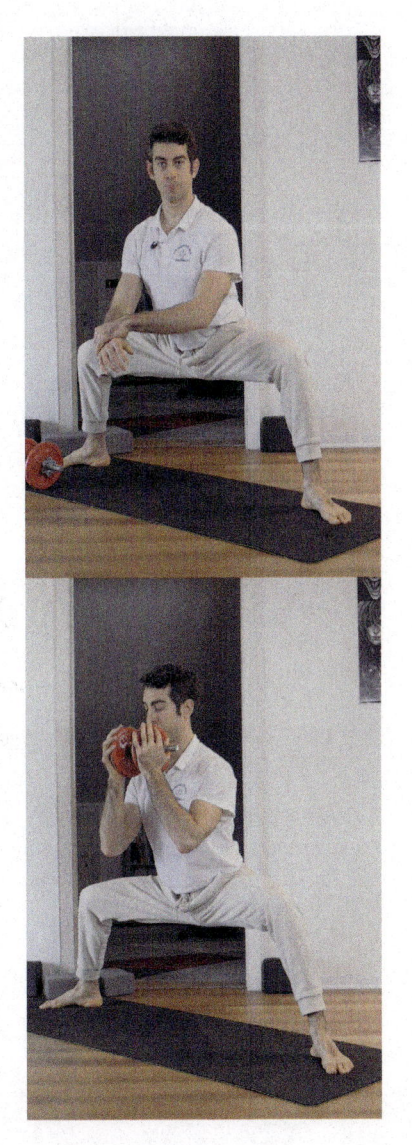

- A **PNF contraction** is possible here, and it's obtained by pushing the knees against the pressure of the hands. Hold the contraction 10 to 20", then release. After the contraction, inhale, exhale, and get deeper into the stretching position, trying to widen the legs more and lower down the hips. Always feel those *glutes* working hard to push your knees out, especially after each PNF contraction.

- **Use a weight**: let it help you push your hips deeper and deeper towards the floor. If you use a weight, I suggest you perform some dynamic repetitions (start standing and go down into a squat), usually 6 to 10, pausing at the bottom of each rep for a couple of seconds before coming back up. At the last repetition, pause a little longer in the stretch, like 5 to 10 breaths.

- **Pull down**: grab a weight on the floor with your hands and push your hips down. This is similar to the previous variation with the weight, but a huge advantage here is that you can adjust the intensity of the stretch as you want.

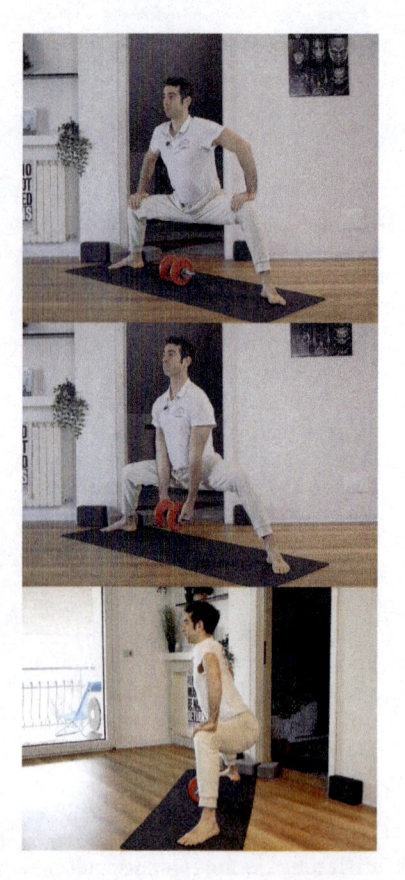

Drive your **knees out**.

Push your **hips down** below your knees' level.

Use different strategies to get deeper into the stretch.

ONE-LEG SQUAT OPENER

This is a wonderful exercise to start working on your squat and, more generally, on your hip abduction range of motion. The reason why you should develop a good squat as a beginner is that the squat is a position that requires good hip and legs flexibility, much similar to the one required in a pancake stretch. Even though the squat is way easier to reach, it's still a very good basic exercise to start with if you want to get serious about the pancake.

Start by placing one foot on a bench by your side. Externally rotate that foot and push the working leg's knee (the one on the bench) strongly out. The foot on the floor must point in front of you with that leg straight at all times. Anterior pelvic tilt, straighten the lower and middle back and fold your torso down slightly more towards the bent leg.

To adjust the intensity of the stretch as you like, you have **two main options**: you can either use a weight or pull yourself into the position using your arms' strength.

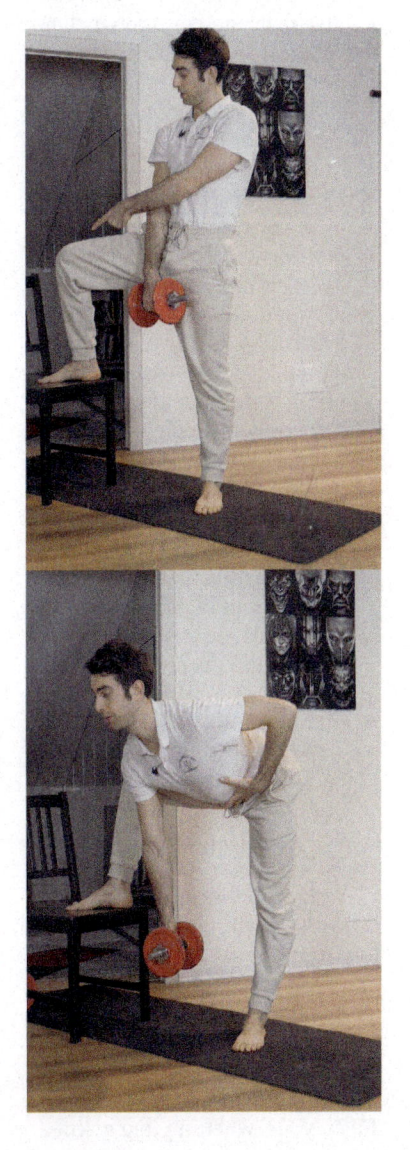

Both are very good strategies to gain more range of motion, and I think that one isn't better than the other. It just depends on the context. During this stretch, you can use two strategies to gain more range of motion.

▸ **Passive static stretch**. Stay in the stretch, trying to reach the deepest position possible by folding your torso in between your legs. Use some **yoga blocks** as a target to understand how deep you're going into the stretch. You can apply a **PNF contraction** by pushing the knee of the working leg against your hand's or elbow's resistance for a count of 10 to 20 seconds. When you stop the contraction, inhale, relax, and on the exhale, try to get a bit deeper into the stretch.

▸ **Dynamic stretch**. From the standing position, fold the torso down, stay in the bottom position for a couple of seconds and come back. This is best done using a weight. I suggest you start with the dynamic variation for 6/8 reps, then on the last rep, stop in the bottom position and stay there, relaxing and applying 1 to 2 PNF contractions.

Push your **working leg's knee** out at all times.

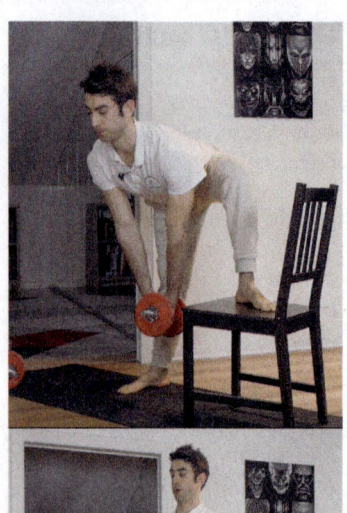

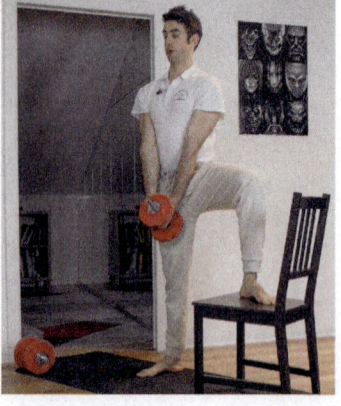

> Put a foot on a support.
>
> Keep your **leg bent**, and **fold you body** in between the legs.
>
> Start with **dynamic reps** and finish with a **passive static** stretch.

COSSACK SQUAT

The cossack squat is one of the best hip openers and one of my favorite exercises to warm up my hips and legs before an intense stretching practice. Start with your legs spread wide apart (like in a horse stance) and squat down toward one leg following these steps:

▸ Drive the knee of the working leg (the one you're squatting on) outwards. *Emphasize* this movement. Engage your glutes.

▸ Keep the **opposite leg straight** and **turn your straight leg's foot up** to simplify the exercise.

▸ Keep your torso upright as much as you can.

▸ Don't lift the working leg's heel off the floor.

Gently drive your hips down following the points written above, and go into the deepest stretch you can handle. The **depth** of your cossack squat strongly depends on your flexibility level: always remember to squat down only until you can maintain a good technique!

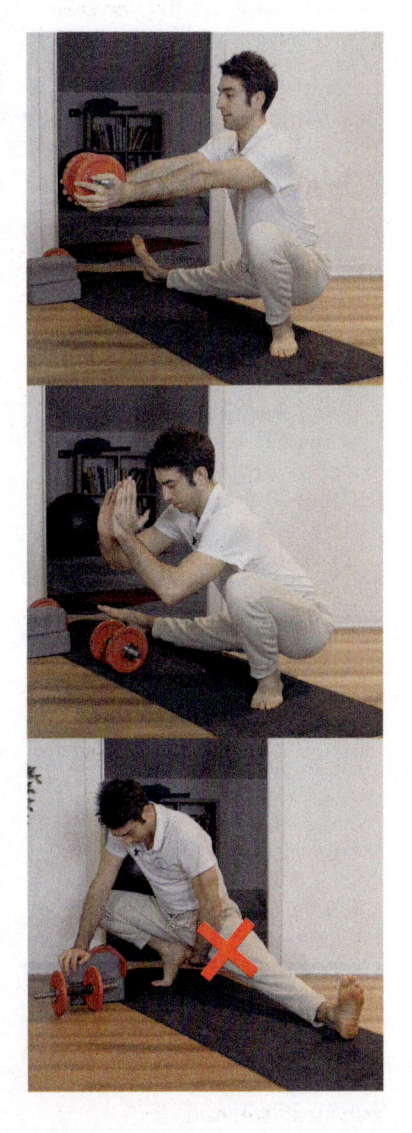

Here are a few strategies you can use to simplify the position and get deeper into the cossack squat position.

▸ **Hold a weight in front of you**. This will counterbalance the weight of your trunk, allowing you to maintain a good *upright torso* positioning.

If you don't have a weight, you can put your hands on something in front of you, like a chair, to help you. **Place something under your working leg's foot**. It should be something sufficiently high, between 10 to 30 cm. By raising that foot, you have to cover less distance to get into the bottom cossack squat position; hence you need less range of motion. When your working leg's foot is higher than the straight leg one, the flexibility demand from your hips is much less.

So far, we've seen how to go into the cossack squat with the correct technique and how to use some strategies to **simplify** the exercise a little bit: I strongly suggest you use them if the cossack squat done on the floor feels like a nightmare, your heel wants to pop off the floor, and you can't maintain a proper technique.

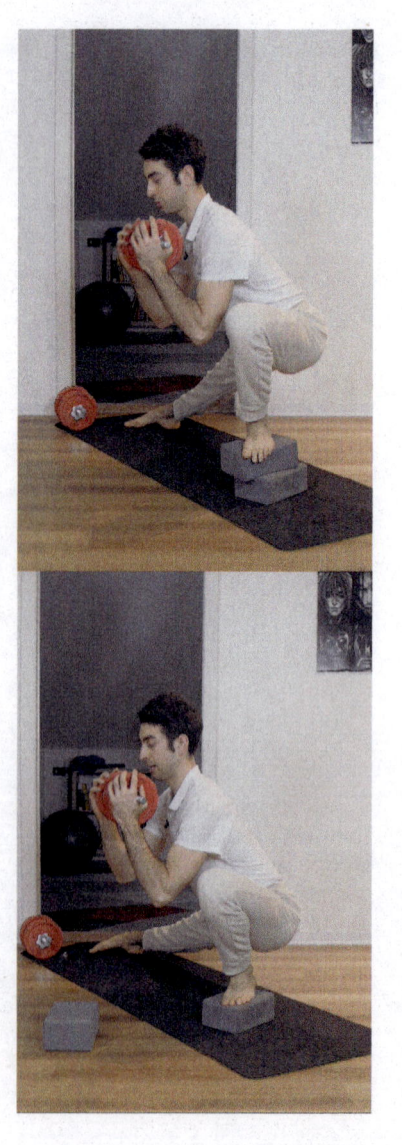

Once you're able to perform the cossack on the floor with a good technique, different variations can **increase your range of motion** and get deeper into the stretch.

- **Isometrics**: stay in the bottom cossack squat position and increase your range of motion there, driving your hips closer and closer to the floor.

- **Dynamic movements**: shift from one leg to the other dynamically, trying to maintain your **hips as low as you can**.

  This is one of my favorite strategies since you can really focus on the hips' abduction and range of motion. Be careful and move slowly.

  At first, when you perform the *transition* from one side to the other, you want to assist the movement by putting your hands on the floor in front of you: this is going to give you much more stability and control during the entire transition and help you with the balance as well.

- As you get better, slowly release the hands until you can do the exercise without any kind of assistance.

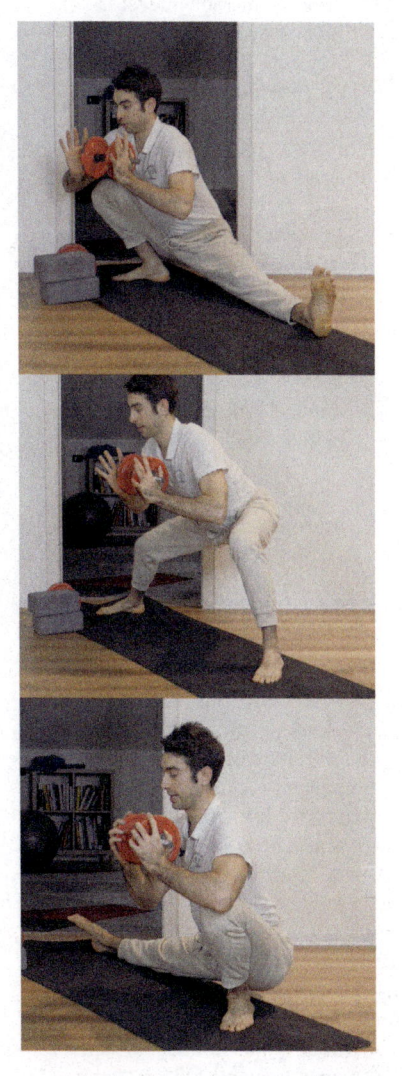

▶ At that point, you can even hold a weight in front of you to further increase the intensity of the stretch. Repeat the transition for reps, usually 8 to 16.

▶ **PNF**: place your elbow against the bent leg's knee and push it out. This will give you an extra *adductors* stretch. Push with the knee against the elbow to obtain a **PNF contraction**, hold it for 10 to 20", then stop, inhale, and try to push your knee further out on the exhale.

As you can see, the cossack squat has really many variations. Start with the one you're more comfortable with and move up from there.

If you're a beginner, I suggest you start with the variation with a block under your working leg's foot and build flexibility there using dynamic repetitions with a weight, pausing for 3 to 4" at the bottom of each rep and for a little longer, like 10 to 20" on the last one.

With time, work on the dynamic variation on the floor until you feel comfortable doing it without your hands' assistance. At an advanced stage, I suggest using the cossack squat as a *warm-up* exercise.

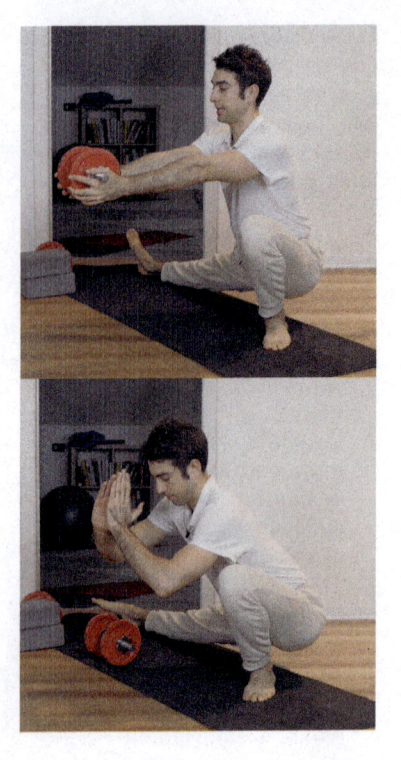

Drive the working leg's **knee out**.

Keep the **opposite leg straight**.

Use different **strategies** to gain range of motion.

90/90 STRETCH

The 90/90 stretch is an excellent stretch for your entire hip joint that allows you to work on your hip *internal* and *external* rotation, on the flexibility of the *ligaments* that stay deep inside of your hips, and on your *glutes* and *piriformis* flexibility as well.

Start sitting on the floor and spread your legs wide apart, keeping your knees flexed, forming a 90° angle. Try to sit down with an anterior pelvic tilt, with your butt pushed back and the base of the hamstrings in contact with the floor as much as you can.

From this position, move your legs laterally, driving one leg out and the other in. For example, drive the right leg down towards your right side and touch the floor with its outer part. Simultaneously, drive the left leg towards your right side until you can touch the floor with your left knee.

During this movement, keep your trunk oriented forward without rotating it to the side.

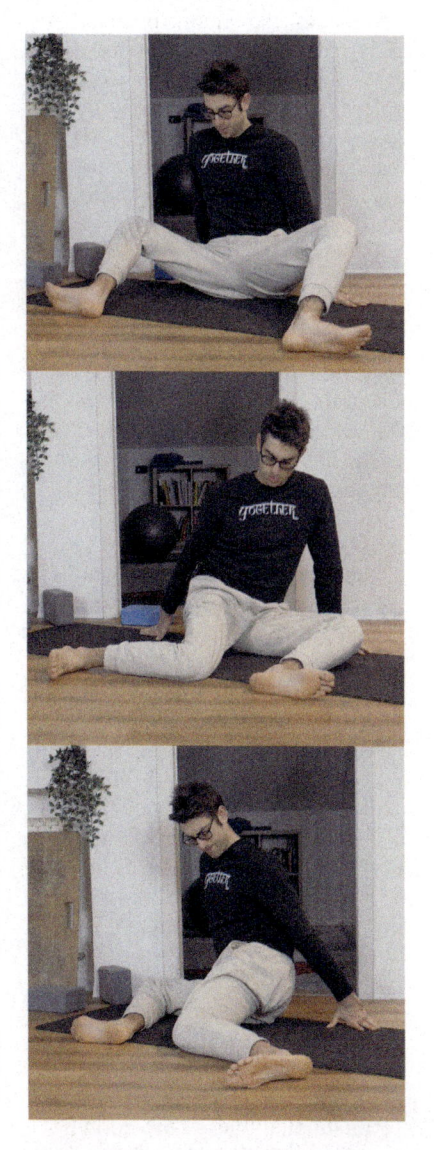

You should finish with both knees on the floor, one leg externally rotated in front of you, and the other one internally rotated, precisely by your side. This is the 90/90 position. Your front hip must stay in contact with the floor, or if you can't touch the floor with it yet, put a yoga block or a pillow under it. The other hip will probably pop out the floor: that's completely fine, especially for men. By the way, do your best to push it down. To create a good stretch effect in a 90/90 position, you have various options.

▸ **Dynamic movements**: during this variation, you want to move your legs towards one side and the other. Start in the center, drive your legs towards one side, spend a couple of seconds there, and then change sides. You'll finish in the exact same position but on the opposite side. Repeat this kind of movement for the desired amount of reps, usually 10 to 15.

▸ **Side leg's hip external rotators stretch**: move your body very gently towards the leg on the side. Try to push that leg's hip down toward the floor (don't overdo it!).

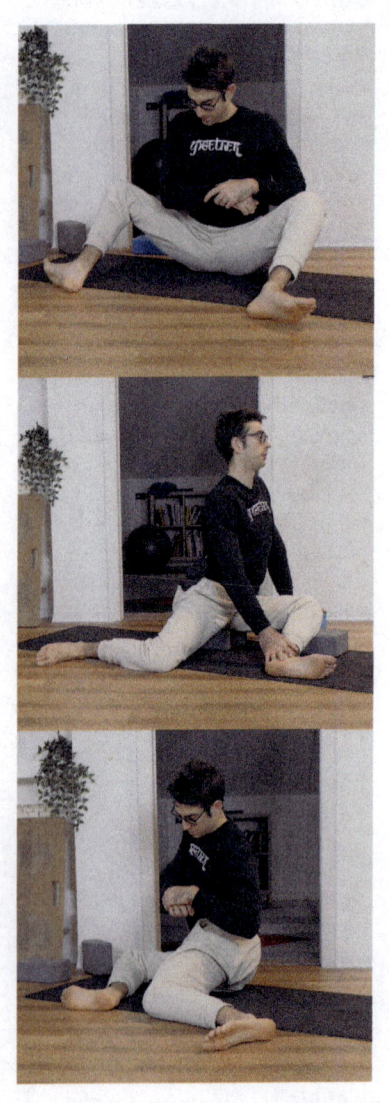

Put a pillow under your back hip to provide extra assistance.

▸ **90/90 lifts**. This strategy improves your **hip internal rotation** and stretches your *hip external rotators*. Now, you may wonder why focusing on the external or internal rotators is so important. This is because these muscles here, if tight, may severely limit **whichever** movement your hips want to perform since they're so deep inside your hip and involved in every hip movement you perform. Having them flexible and strong is a must, much like the muscles of the rotator's cuff in the shoulder. To perform this exercise, once you have rotated to the side, rotate your body as well toward your front leg. From there, you want to keep your torso as upright as possible, your hips still, and you want to lift your back foot up as much as possible. It's probably going to move just a little. That's fine: it's supposed to be like that. That's a short range!

At each point of the transition you want to make sure you're pushing your knees **one away from the other**.

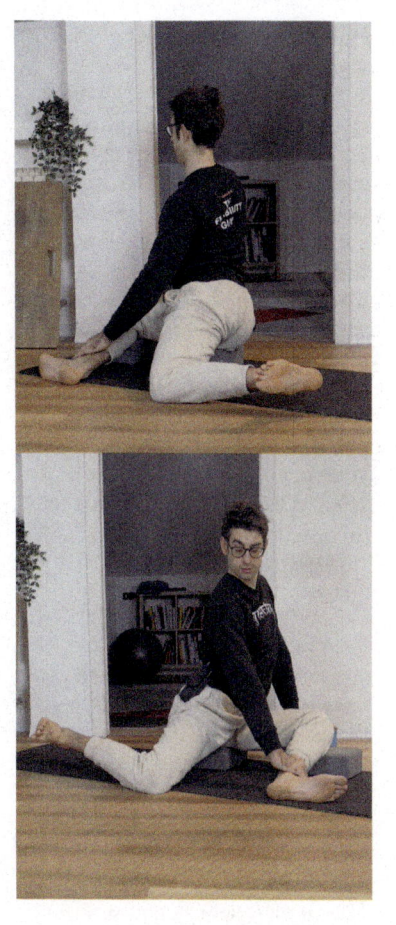

> Keep your **knees as wide as possible** as you perform the transitions.
>
> Different variations are possible to stretch your entire hip joint.

PIGEON POSE

When you perform a 90/90 stretch, there's the point where you move your legs to the side, and you have one leg in front of you, bent at 90°, and one back, bent at 90° as well. This can be the starting position of a wonderful *glute* and *piriformis* stretch: the **pigeon pose**.

First, if this position feels uncomfortable to you, you can put some yoga blocks under your front hip and front knee to raise your body a little higher: this will create a little less stretch, making the position possible to practice.

Keeping your front leg bent at 90° and your trunk oriented toward that direction, you want to extend your **back leg** and **internally rotate it**. Thinking about facing down with your back knee and foot may help you understand how to internally rotate that back leg. This is going to create a strong stretching effect on your *glutes* and *piriformis* muscles. The most important thing you have to think about in order to create a good stretch is pushing your back hip (the one of the extended leg) down toward the floor. By doing so, you'll create more rotation on your hips, and that rotation is what creates and intensifies the stretch here.

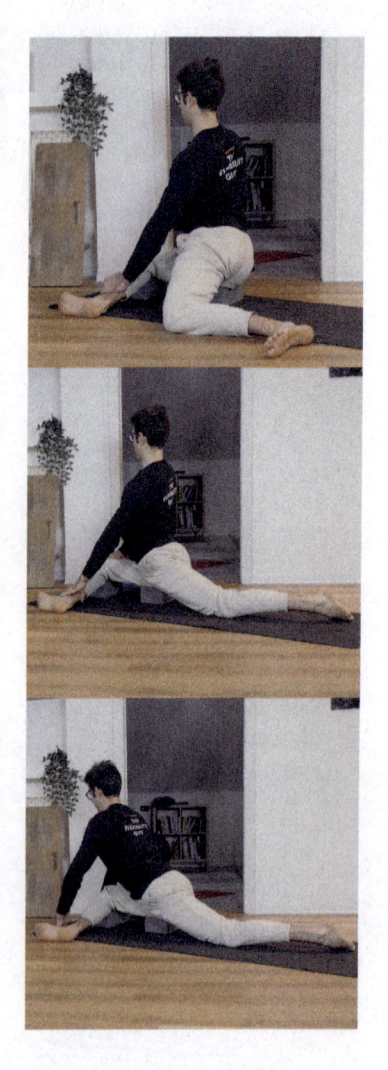

You can use two **stretching methodologies**.

▸ **Passive static stretching**. Stay in the stretch, drive your back hip down, internally rotate your back leg, and get deeper and deeper into the stretch. You can apply a PNF contraction during the passive static position: push your front foot against the floor for 10 to 15", then stop, inhale, and on the exhale, try to get deeper into the stretch.

▸ You can do a **dynamic stretch** by driving your torso down toward the front leg and coming back up. As you do so, remember that you want to push your back hip down and keep your back as straight as possible.

In order to get deeper in the stretch, you have **three main options**.

The first is **squaring** your hips more and more.

The **second** is folding your trunk toward your front leg.

The **third** is moving your hips closer to the floor. Remove the yoga blocks from under your hips and front knee and get deeper into the stretch.

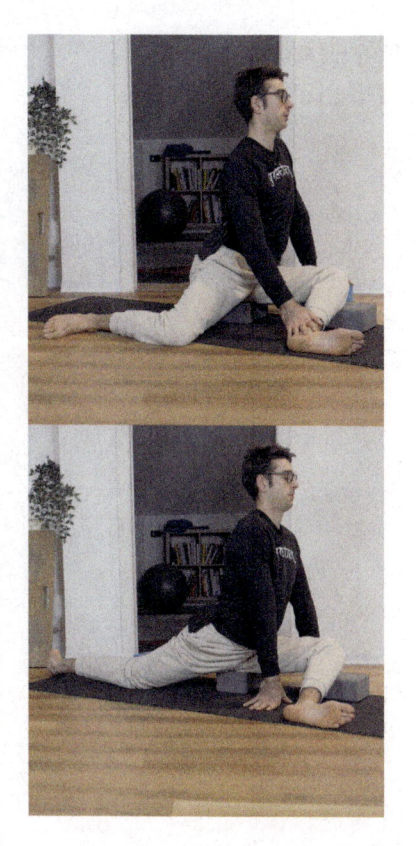

> Keep your front knee bent at 90° or a little less.
>
> Extend and internally rotate your back leg as much as you can.
>
> **PNF**: push your front foot against the floor.

LYING GLUTES AND PIRIFORMIS

Another really strong and excellent *glutes* and *piriformis* stretch. Start by lying with your back on the floor with your feet on a wall, and take 30/40 centimeters away from the wall with your butt.

Now, place one foot in contact with the other leg, slightly below the knee level: you need to externally rotate that leg in order to do this kind of movement, and that will be the working leg.

At this point, slowly bend the other leg (the one you have against the wall), bringing that knee towards your chest. Don't lift your glutes off the floor as you do that, and assist the traction with your hands if needed. As you do this, push the knee of the working leg away from you toward the wall.

The closer your knee gets to your chest, the harder the exercise will be. Ideally, to obtain a really strong stretch, you want to arch your lower back a little.

If the stretch gets easy, move your hips closer and closer to the wall. Keep in mind, though, that you don't want to lift your lower back off the floor.

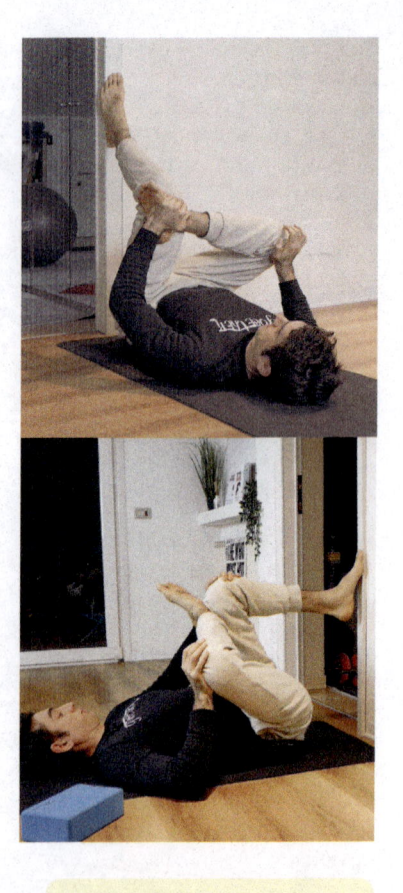

> Don't lift your lower back off the floor.
>
> **PNF**: push the working leg's foot agains the opposite knee.

CALF STRETCHES

Calves are really important muscles to stretch if you want to have a flexible lower body and achieve the pancake stretch. To refresh your ideas, this is because they play a role during knee flexion (bending the knee), and, quite on the opposite, what we want during a pancake is having our knees completely straight.

To perform this exercise, put one foot on some yoga blocks, keeping your knee completely straight. You want to incline the foot as needed to feel a deep sensation of stretch, moving your heel as close as possible to the blocks. The stretch is created by gently moving your body forward and leaning on your front foot. The more you do that, the harder the stretch.

To make the exercise even more intense, move your trunk and put your hands on something, like a chair or similar object (I'm using a fit ball here), and continue leaning on your front foot.

As you perform this exercise, keep in mind that you want to maintain a straight lower back position and both of your legs straight, putting particular attention on your front leg.

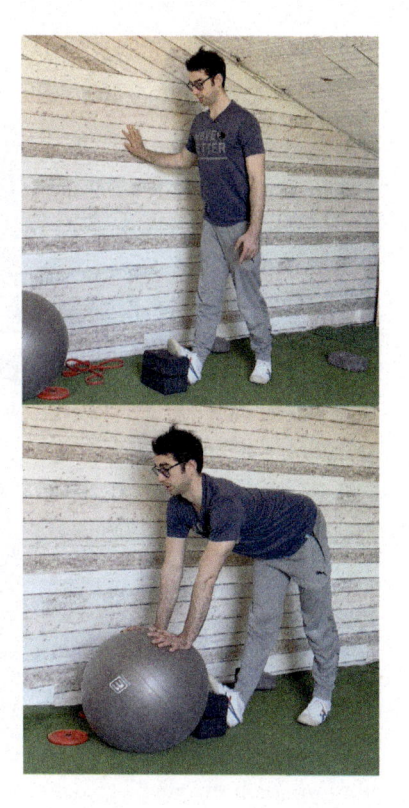

Use 1 or 2 yoga blocks under your front toe.

Load the front leg to increase the stretch.

PNF: push the ball of your front foot down.

TAILOR POSE

This is a wonderful exercise you can use to stretch your *adductors* and *pubofemoral ligaments* with a movement that combines **hip abduction, flexion, and external rotation**. Some of you might find this exercise quite easy to perform, but I highly recommend to those of you who do struggle with this one to use it to improve your general hip joint's flexibility.

Start in a seated position with your back against a wall and the soles of your feet together in front of your hips. The closer your feet are to your hips, the harder the exercise will be. From here, the aim of the stretch is to push your knees down toward the floor until you can eventually reach it. As you do so, make sure to:

- **Press your knees down with your hands**. Keep your hands on your knees and push them down to create the stretch.

- Put **weights on the knees** (if you have some weights available) in order to make the stretch even more intense.

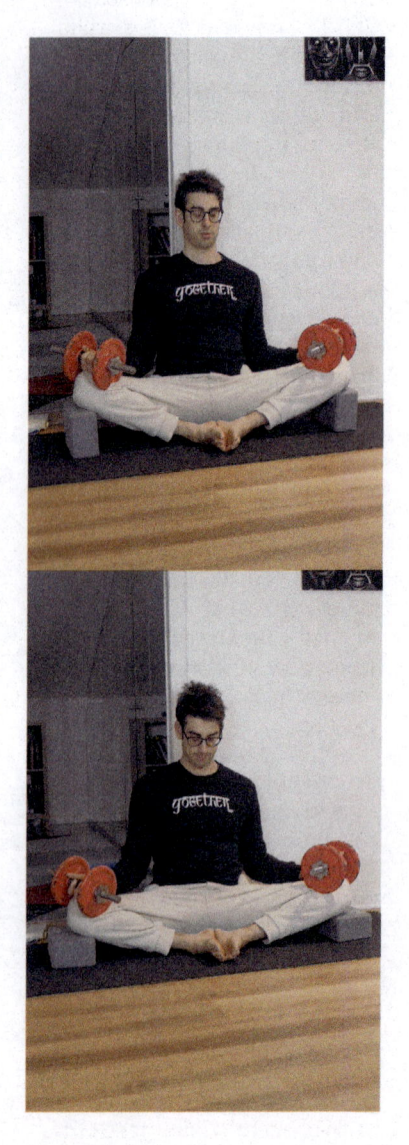

Throughout the stretch, you want to stay with your back and glutes as close to the wall as possible, but please take note that coming a little bit away from it is completely normal: don't worry about it.

Since the purpose of this stretch is touching the floor with your knees, I strongly suggest you place some yoga blocks under your knees to relax better in your max range of motion and keep track of your progress. As you are in the stretch, you want to gently press your knees against the yoga blocks: as you can really apply pressure on them, you know that it's time for a change, and you can get deeper into the stretch.

You can use two **stretching methodologies**.

1) **PNF**: push your knees up against the weights and/or hands resistance.

2) Use **PNF and antagonist contraction** together for reps: push your knees up during the PNF just for a brief moment, like 2 or 3 seconds, then, immediately after, push them strongly down towards the floor, squeezing your glutes. Repeat for the desired number of reps (10 to 20).

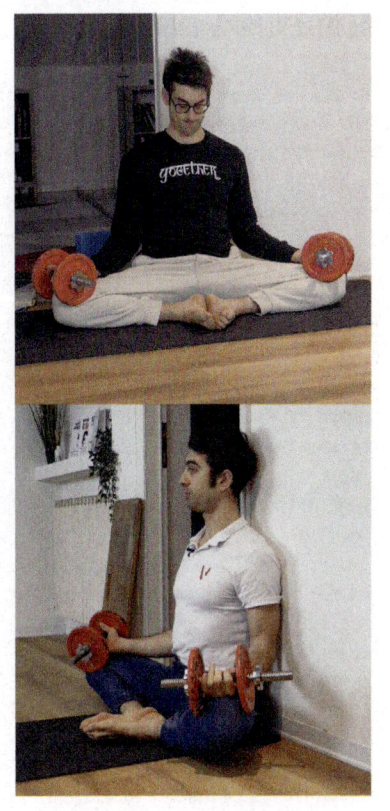

> Keep the soles of your feet in front of your hips.
>
> Drive your **knees down** using weights and/or hands assistance.
>
> Combine **PNF** and **antagonist contractions**.

53

KNEELING ONE LEG PIKE

Sit down on a bench with one leg on it, and the other leg bent with the knee on the floor. The leg which remains on the bench is the stretched leg. If you don't have a bench, don't worry: use two chairs instead. Make sure to place the bottom leg correctly: put some yoga blocks under the knee and drive it slightly back, creating pressure on the blocks. If this feels uncomfortable, put the leg in front of you, with your foot on the floor. That's an easier way to do this stretch. Make sure that the stretched leg's hip is well pressed against the bench for the whole duration of the stretch. Now, three main variations are possible.

▸ **Bent leg.** This is the easiest variation, and I strongly suggest you start with this one. Keep your working leg bent with your knee in contact with your chest and extend it as long as your chest remains in contact with your knee. Grab your front knee with one arm in order to keep your trunk pressed toward your leg, and with the other arm grab the bench to pull yourself even further into the stretch.

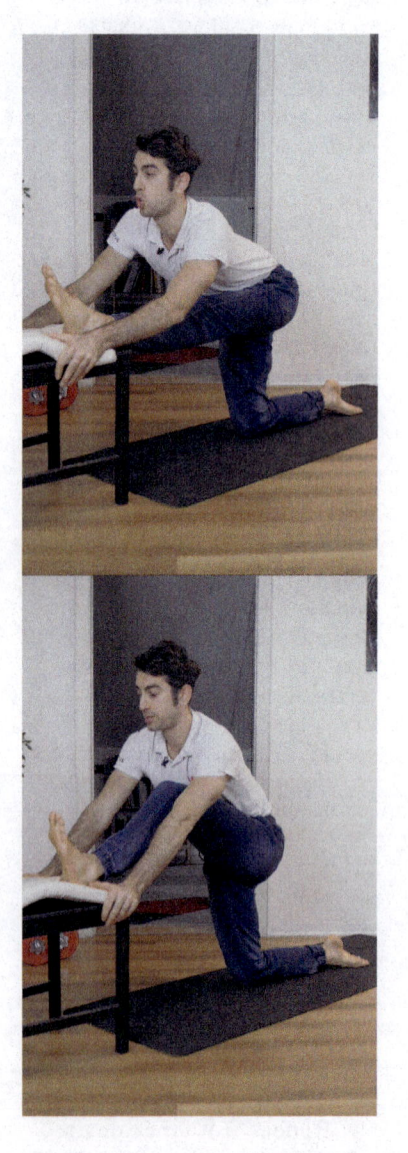

- **Straight leg.** The concept here is the same as for the bent leg variation, except that the working leg has to be straight at all times during the stretch. Fold your trunk towards your front leg, keeping the knee completely straight until you can feel the desired amount of stretch on your hip extensors.

- **Dynamic.** This is a combination between the bent leg and the straight leg variations.
Start in the bent leg variation and reach your max stretch with your chest in contact with the knee. Once there, without moving your trunk at all, straighten the working leg completely, remain in the straight-leg variation for a few seconds, and come back in the bent-leg one. Repeat for reps.

Remember to keep your lower & middle back **straight**. Drive your head forward: this helps you maintain your lower and middle back in the correct position and further increase the stretch.

To intensify the stretch, you can grab the bench and pull yourself forward, or you can grab a weight with one hand and let it pull your body down.

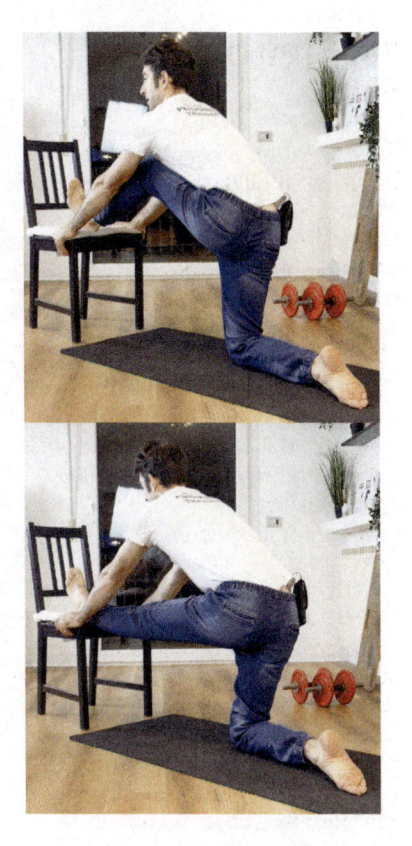

One leg on the bench (or chairs), one knee on the floor.

PNF: push your front heel against the bench or pull your trunk away from your front leg (bent leg variation only).

SEATED ONE LEG PIKE

Sit down on a bench with one leg on it and the other one down. The leg that stays on the bench will be the stretched leg. Despite that, it's still important to put the other leg in the correct manner: place some blocks under the free leg's knee and drive it slightly back, creating pressure with it on the blocks. Make also sure to press down the hip of the stretched leg against the bench. Two variations are possible:

▸ **Bent leg**: chest in contact with the knee, trying to straighten the front leg as much as you can. The most important thing is that the chest remains in contact with the knee.

▸ **Straight leg**: completely extend the knee and fold the trunk toward the front leg. Keep the front leg completely straight.

▸ **Dynamic**: mix the bent and straight leg variation extending and bending the leg for reps, trying to push the chest down at all times.

Doesn't matter the variation; keep your back straight and push your head forward.

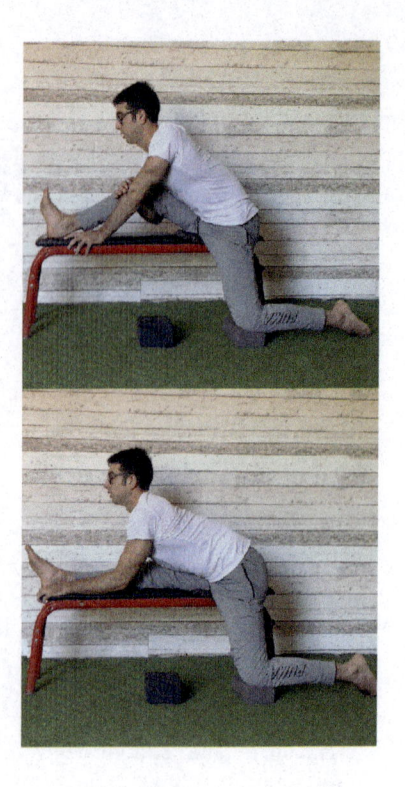

> Keep your back straight and push your head forward.
>
> **PNF**: push your front heel down.
>
> **Antagonist**: squeeze your quads and lift your front foot up.

ONE LEG STANDING PIKE

Make a lunge, turn the back foot out at 45°, and point your front foot forward. From this position, there are two main variations possible.

First variation: bend the front leg and drive the body down until your chest enters in contact with your front knee. Wrap your front knee with the arm on the same side and, keeping the contact between your chest and the knee at all times, straighten the front leg until you can feel the desired sensation of stretch.

In the **second variation,** the technique remains exactly the same, only this time, you want to completely straighten your front knee and move your body down from there. Here it doesn't matter how far you can go into the stretch: the most important thing is that your front leg remains straight.

In both variations, a really useful thing you can think about is driving your head in front of you (and not toward the leg) and moving your hips into anterior pelvic tilt as much as possible.

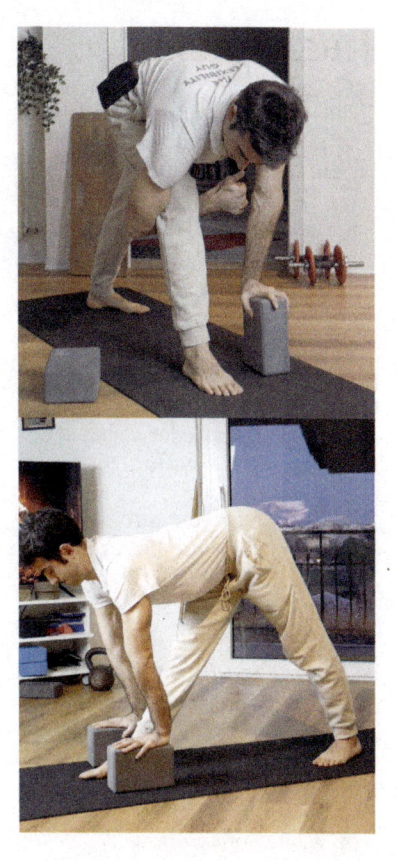

> Bent leg variation: keep your chest in contact with the knee.
>
> Straight leg variation: keep your front leg straight.
>
> **PNF**: push your front heel against the floor.

FROG STRETCH

This is one of my favorites exercises to develop terrific **hip abduction flexibility**.
Start lying on your back with your feet against a wall and your lower back slightly arched. Keep a 90° angle on your knees and between your legs and trunk, which means that your knees should be in line with your hips if watched from above, and your knees have to be in line with your hips.

Now, to create the stretch, you want to **push your knees down** toward the floor. The only strength of your arms won't be sufficient, though, so you have two options. You can either grab some weights with your hands and put the weights and your hands on your knees, or you can wrap some weights around your knees, using a band or whatever you want. Both work well.

The concept of **wrapping the weights** around your knees is the best choice, in my opinion, as they pull your knees down with the best assistance they can provide, as you won't be forced to hold them with your hands.

By the way, if you can find a good set-up and activations holding the weights with your hands on top of your knees, that's a good alternative too!

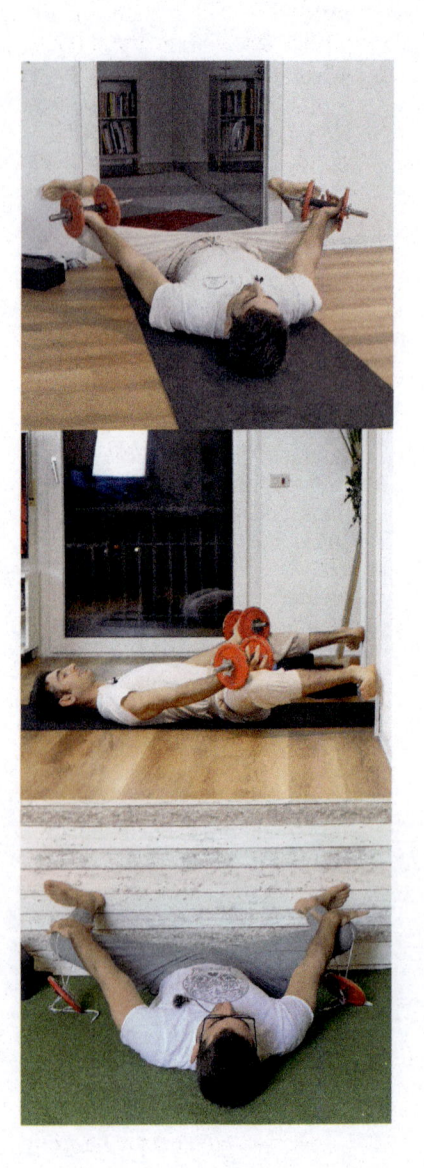

Remember to start with a weight you can control and that helps you get deeper into the stretch. Usually, I suggest starting with 3/4 kgs per side. Remember, though, that the weights shouldn't do all the job: you have to **use your hands to push down the knees** even more if needed.

Relax your adductors and hips, and as you gain more and more range of motion, let the knees get closer and closer to the floor. Remember, though, to keep your feet in line with your knees at all times! Not higher nor lower. For instance, if you move your knees further towards the floor, move your feet too!

You can use two techniques to increase your range of motion:

▸ **PNF**: **push your knees up** against the weights' resistance and the pressure of your hands. Hold that contraction for 10 to 20", then relax, inhale, place your hands under the knees to relax a bit the legs, exhale, and try to get deeper into the stretch.

▸ Keep always an **antagonist contraction** on your glutes, squeezing your muscles as if you wanted to separate your legs even more.

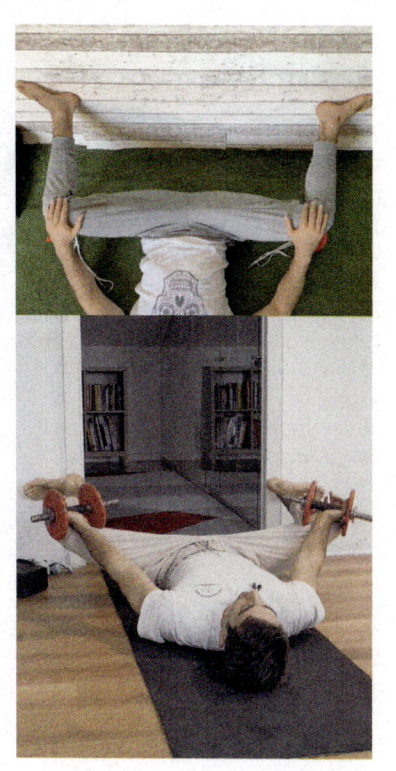

Put some **weights** on your knees.

Keep a 90° angle on the knees and between your trunk and legs.

Use **PNF**, **antagonist contractions** and a mix of both.

COMPASS HIP OPENER

This is an extremely interesting exercise to increase your hip abduction flexibility. Now, make sure to understand the starting position of this stretch, as it's a little complicated, but as soon as you get it, the exercise is really simple in itself.

Start in a lunge and turn your back in, flexing your knee at 90°. Now, turn your body towards the back leg until you have your trunk parallel to the legs. From here, start with your hips far away from the floor, then drive them down toward the floor, more precisely **toward the front leg's heel**. Aim for your max range of motion, remain for a couple of seconds in the bottom position and come back to the starting position. During the entire movement, try not to move your legs: they have to stay in the exact same position for the whole duration of the exercise. Remember to **anterior pelvic tilt**: arch your lower back a little as you perform this exercise.

You need to feel the stretch both on the *hamstrings* and *glutes* of the front leg and on the back leg's *adductors*. Push your hips forward and keep them squared.

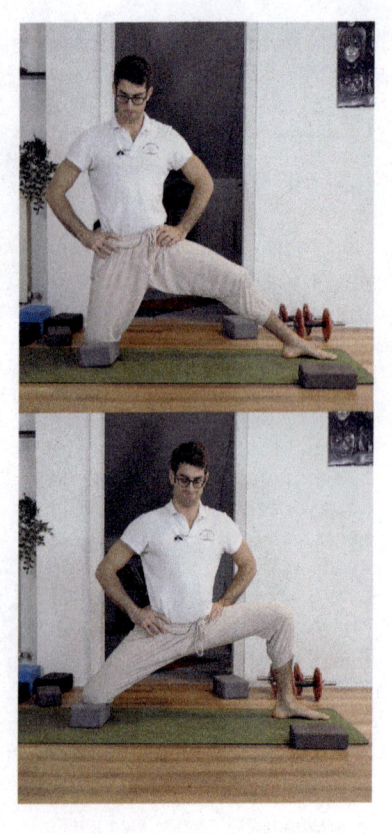

> Drive your **hips down** towards the front leg's heel.
>
> Remain for 2" at the bottom of each rep.
>
> **PNF**: push your back leg's knee against the floor.

WALL HAMSTRINGS AND CALVES

This is a wonderful exercise that stretches your hamstrings and calves deeply with one single movement. First, place one foot against a wall, with the heel as close to the wall as possible and the sole in contact with the wall. If you are a beginner, start by placing your heel slightly away from the wall. Then, as you get better and better, move it closer.

Keep your hips as squared as possible as you perform the stretch: the front leg's hip must be pulled back, and the back leg's hip pushed forward. Also, remember that your back knee should stay exactly under your back leg's hip, as shown.

From this position, fold your torso down towards your front leg and try to reach the wall with your head keeping your lower and middle back as straight as possible until you feel the desired amount of stretch on your front leg.

Different progressions are possible, depending on your flexibility level: hands on the wall (beginner), hands on some yoga blocks or on the floor (intermediate), and chest to the knee (advanced).

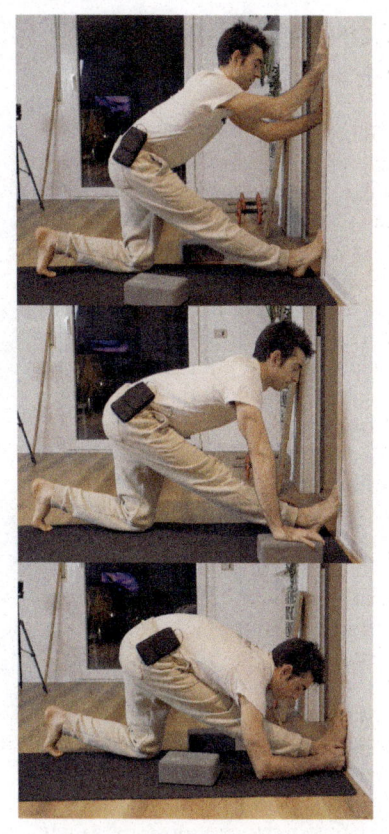

> Keep your front leg straight.
>
> Maintain your hips as squared as possible.
>
> **PNF**: push your front heel against the floor and your toe against the wall at the same time.

61

ONE LEG PIKE EXTENSION

This is an excellent loaded stretching exercise for your hip extensors and calves.

From a standing position, grab a weight, like a barbell on your back or a dumbbell, with your hands. Move one leg in front of you, putting your front toe on some yoga blocks. Turn your back foot out 45° to ensure good stability in the position.

From there, fold your trunk down towards your front leg, keeping your hips squared (right hip in line with the left hip) and your lower and middle back as straight as possible. **Control the way down**: it should last 2 to 4". Reach the best stretch you can handle, stop there for a couple of seconds, and then come back to the starting position *with control*. That's one repetition. Usually, I suggest performing 6 to 10 of these, always controlling the movements at your best.

As this gets easier and easier, raise your front foot up, moving your front leg closer and closer to your trunk.

Use a weight that helps you get deeper and doesn't make you resist to the stretch.

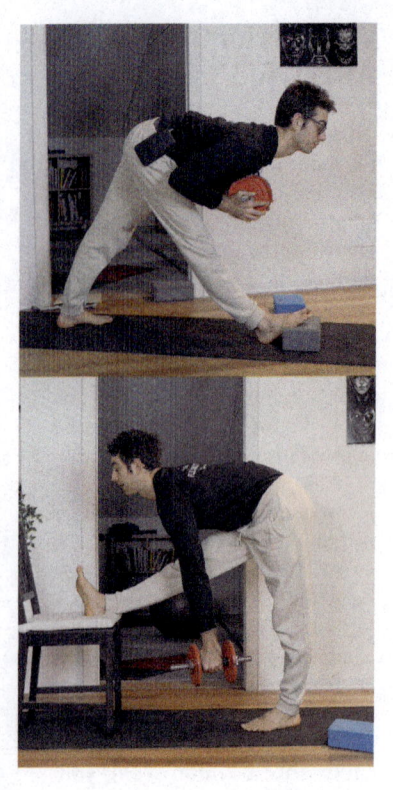

> Keep both legs **straight**.
>
> Maintain your **hips squared** at all times.
>
> Drive your **torso down** and forward towards your front leg until you can feel the desired amount of stretch.

CHEST TO WALL SPLIT

The chest-to-wall split is an excellent exercise to work on your hip abduction with your legs straight, which is exactly what you do in a pancake.

Start sitting on the floor facing a wall. Put your feet against the wall and slowly move your hips closer to it, **spreading your legs apart**. Your knees should remain straight at all times, and your trunk as perpendicular to the floor as possible, even better if a little tilted toward the wall. Move your hips closer and closer to the wall until you can feel the desired amount of stretch. Stop there and relax. To prevent your hips from moving away from the wall, **keep your hands behind your butt**: this will lock your hips in place and let you keep the same amount of stretch throughout the exercise.

To apply a **PNF contraction**, push your feet against the wall for 10 to 20", then stop, inhale, exhale, and try to get deeper into the stretch spreading your feet a little wider.

You can apply an **antagonist contraction** by *squeezing your glutes* as if you wanted to spread your legs even more.

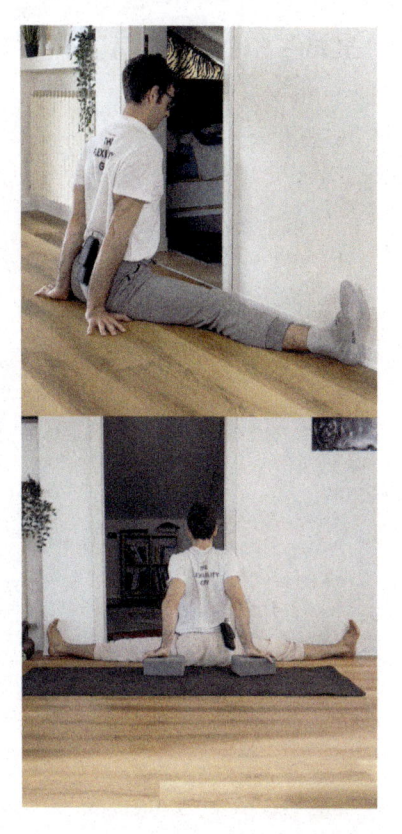

Spread your legs wide apart.

Keep your **hands behind your hips**.

Use **PNF** and a **continuous** antagonist contraction.

LYING SIDE SPLIT

This is a fantastic exercise for your legs apart flexibility, hence for your pancake stretch as well. Start lying with your back on the floor, your butt against a wall, and your legs completely straight. You can arch a little bit your lower back. Put some weights on your feet or on your knees. Do you remember the distinction I made between these two strategies during the frog pose? Here it works exactly the same.

- You can **wrap some weights around your feet**, and to do so, I suggest you use some ankle weights or weights with some bands wrapped around them.

- Otherwise, you can put the **weights on your knees** and keep them there with your hands.

Keeping your legs in contact with the wall, slide down with your feet, spreading your legs as wide as possible. Remember to keep your legs straight at all times and your feet pointing back: this will ensure a bit of external rotation on your legs, which helps you find a better stretch. If you're a beginner, your legs may remain a little bent, but that's fine.

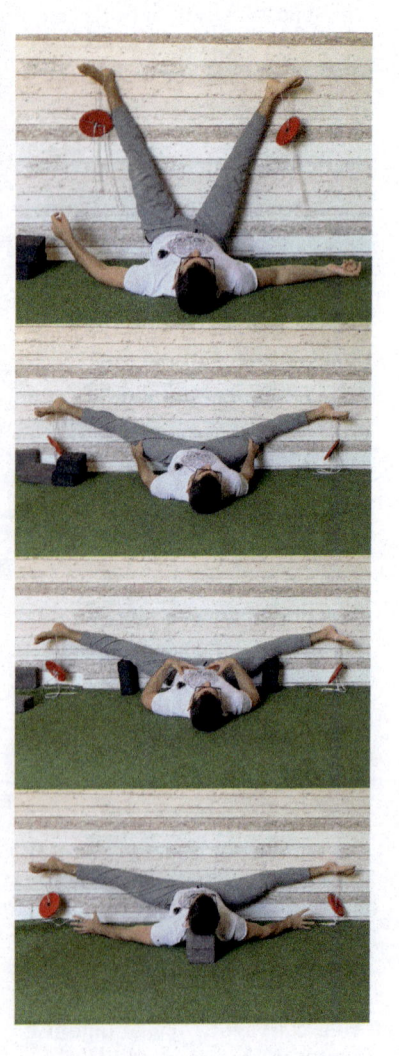

Once in the stretch, you can use different strategies.

- **PNF**. Put your hands on the knees and push your legs up against your hands and weights' resistance. Hold the contraction for 10 to 20". After the PNF contraction, relax your legs by putting your hands under your knees to sustain them, inhale, and on the exhale, stretch deeper.

- **Antagonist contraction**. As you are in the position, *squeeze your glutes* and *push your feet down*. I suggest you use this kind of contraction continuously throughout the exercise to help you better relax in the position. You can also combine an antagonist contraction with a PNF. To do this **badass technique**, push your feet up for 2", then down for another 2". Repeat for 10 to 20 reps, then stop, inhale, exhale, and get deeper.

You can put some yoga blocks under your knees to better relax and keep track of your depth and progress. As you get deeper, move them lower.

You can do this exercise **without a wall**: make sure to keep your legs straight and in line with your hips.

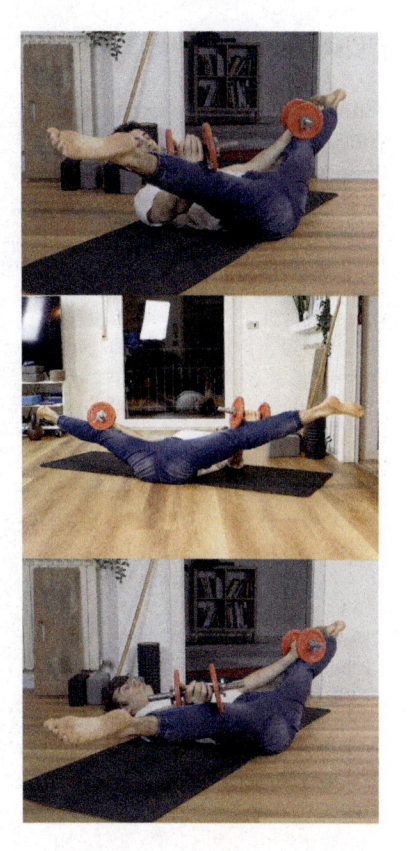

Spread your legs wide apart.

Use some **weights** to **increase** the **intensity** of the stretch.

Use **PNF** and **Antagonist Contractions**.

KNEELING ONE LEG PANCAKE

Start with one knee on the floor and one foot on a chair or a bench by your side. Spread your legs apart as much as possible, or at least more than 90 degrees. At this point, you want to fold your trunk toward the middle of your legs, keeping the leg you have on the bench, the **working leg**, straight at all times.

Put some yoga blocks under your hands as you fold your trunk down to better relax into the stretch and to keep track of your progress. With time, aim to lower the blocks and get deeper into the stretch.

Another interesting variation you can work on is the **lateral pancake variation**. During this variation, rather than flexing your body forward, you want to bend it laterally, as shown in the pictures on this page. Your trunk has to be perpendicular to the floor as you do this, and you can put a yoga block between your trunk and your leg to relax better into the stretch.

Something that may help you here is thinking about putting one shoulder on top of the other: this will give you the idea of placing your trunk perpendicular to the floor.

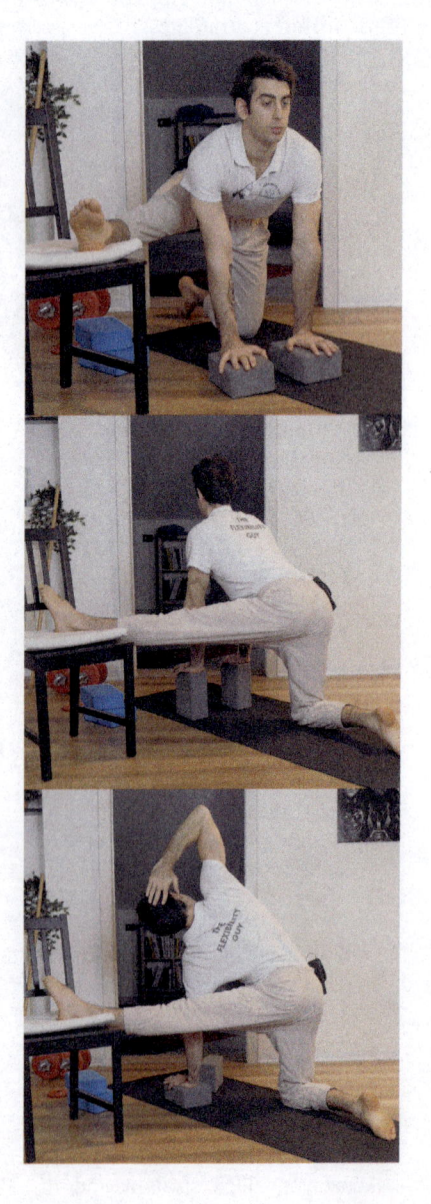

Once the correct technique of this exercise is understood, give the **loaded stretching variations** a go.

To apply a **loaded stretch**, grab a weight with your hands, put it in front of your chest, and fold your trunk toward the middle of your legs. Gently and slowly move your body down, controlling each and every position, pause for a couple of seconds in the deepest stretch you can reach, and come back up. Repeat the movement for reps, and on the final one, remain in the stretch for a little longer, like 5 to 10 breaths.

You can use a **weight** also in the lateral variation, only this time, rather than keeping the weight in front of your chest, put it behind your head and let it pull your trunk down, or you can also straighten your arm up and let the weight push you down in that way. Both strategies work fine.

A **PNF contraction** can help you gain range of motion during the passive static variation (without the weight). Push your working leg's heel against the support for 10 to 20", then stop, inhale, and on the exhale, get deeper into the stretch.

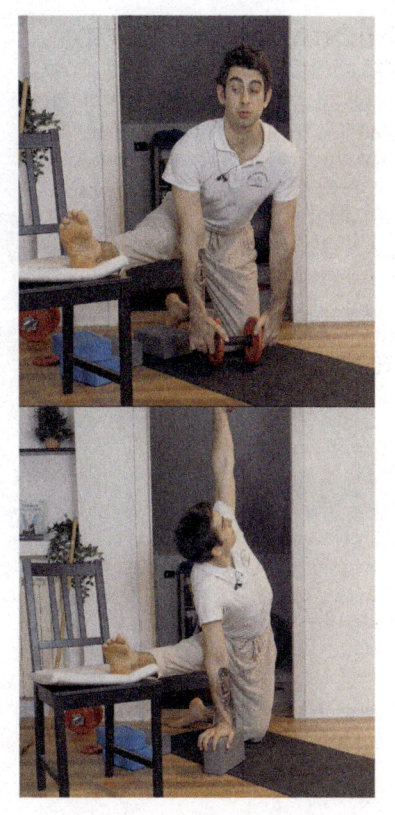

Move your body **in between your legs** (classic variation) or **laterally**.

Use a **weight** to increase the stretch.

PNF: push your heel against the support.

SQUAT MOBILIZATION

The trunk and hip position you use in a squat are really similar to the one you use in a pancake stretch: the "only" difference is that in a pancake your legs are straight, but working in a squat position can really benefit your pancake development.

From a full squat position, you can explore the following movements in order to give your hips a good stretch. If you can't squat fully, don't worry: put some supports under your heels until you can get as deep as you want in the squat.

Push one knee out. Place one hand on the same side's knee and push it out as much as possible. You can repeat this dynamically, or you can stay passively in the position, constantly pushing the knee out.

Push both knees out. Place your elbows against your knees and take your hands together. Push your hands down and your elbows out. This will open your knees out, creating a strong adductors stretch. Again, dynamic and isometric variations are possible.

PNF: push your knee or knees against your hands or elbows.

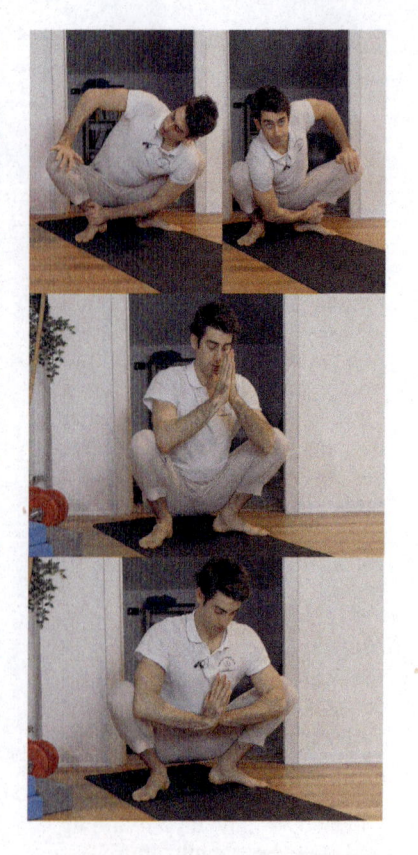

> Start in a **full squat** position.
>
> Push one **knee** or both of your **knees out**.
>
> **PNF**: push your knee or knees against your hands/elbows resistance.

SQUAT OPENER

This is another fantastic exercise you can use to work on your **squat** position, which, as I repeat, is also super important for your pancake development.

Start in a squat position on a support like a bench or two chairs. Turn your feet slightly out and straighten your lower and middle back as much as you can. If you can't stay comfortably in a squat yet, put something under your heels and raise them a bit until you can find your sweet spot.

Take a weight with your hands and drive it down in front of you, letting it go outside of the support, pulling you towards the floor.

Fold your trunk forward and down, following the assistance of the weight, entering the stretching position trying to explore your max range of motion. Spread your legs wide apart, squeezing your glutes to push your knees out as much as you can. As you go down, **try not to lift your butt**: only your trunk should go down. Vice versa, your butt must stay pushed down towards the bench or supports.

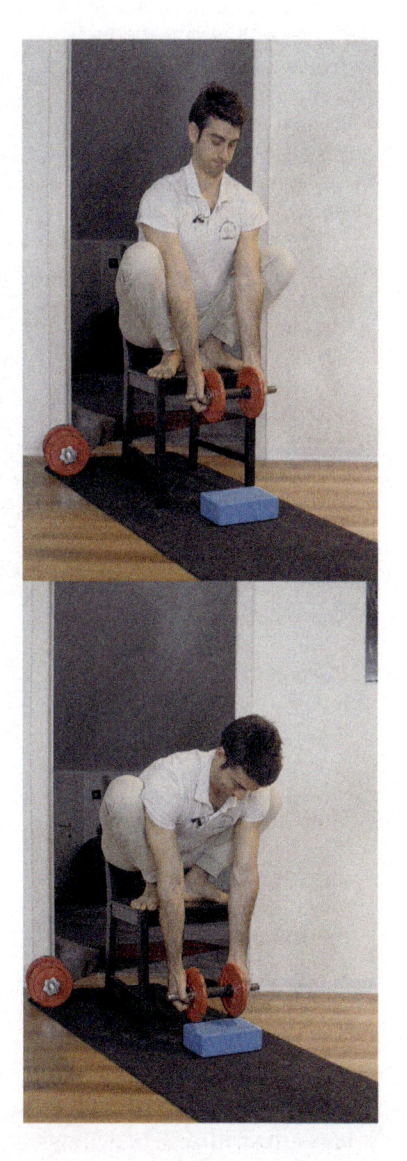

According to your flexibility level, put some yoga blocks on the floor as a target: the higher the blocks, the easier the stretch, and vice versa. Every time you go into the stretch, make sure to touch them with the weight. In this way, you'll be sure to cover the same range of motion every time you go into the stretch and/or remain there. You can use two stretching methodologies.

▸ **Dynamic and passive variations**: from a standard squat position, reach the deepest position possible by driving your trunk down, pause in the bottom position for a brief moment, and come back or remain in the stretch.

▸ **Antagonist contraction**: as you're trying to move your trunk down, *squeeze your glutes* as much as you can, like if you wanted to spread your knees wider apart. Hold the contraction for 10/15", then relax and try to get deeper into the stretch. Repeat 3/5 times.

What you have to prioritize is your **knees' positioning**: it is way better to spread your knees wide apart rather than forcing yourself down, closing your knees inwards. Keep your technique honest at all times.

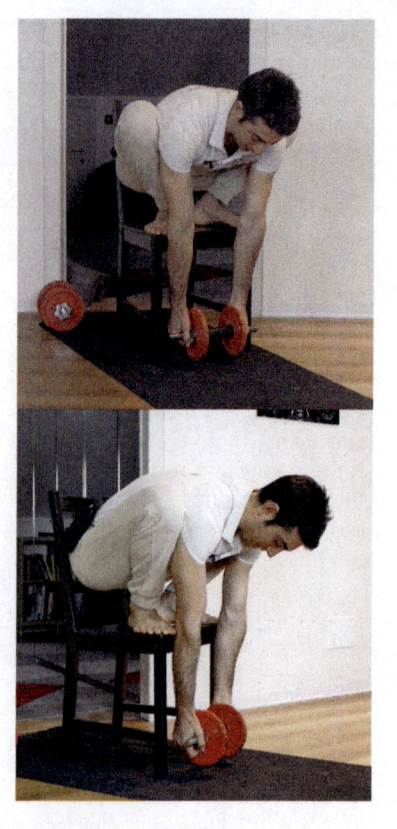

Fold your trunk in between your legs.

Keep your **butt pushed down**.

Different **stretching methodologies** can be applied.

COSSACK PANCAKE

You can further explore the **cossack squat** position flexing your trunk forward to create a strong hips and legs stretch.

Start in the bottom position of a cossack squat position with the straight leg externally rotated (your foot should point up), and your bent leg's knee pushed strongly out. Once there, **fold your trunk forward,** exactly toward the middle of your legs, which isn't exactly in front of you: as you can see in the pictures on this page, I'm driving my trunk **slightly more toward my straight leg**.

Push your head forward during the folding motion and maintain a straight lower and middle back. You can move your trunk in different directions to obtain a slightly different stretch.

Something I suggest you do here is to move your trunk in **different directions**: you can move it *toward your straight leg, toward your bent leg, or in between the legs*. Depending on where you move it, you'll stretch one leg more than the other, and it's totally fine: explore all the ranges of motion available here for the best flexibility gains.

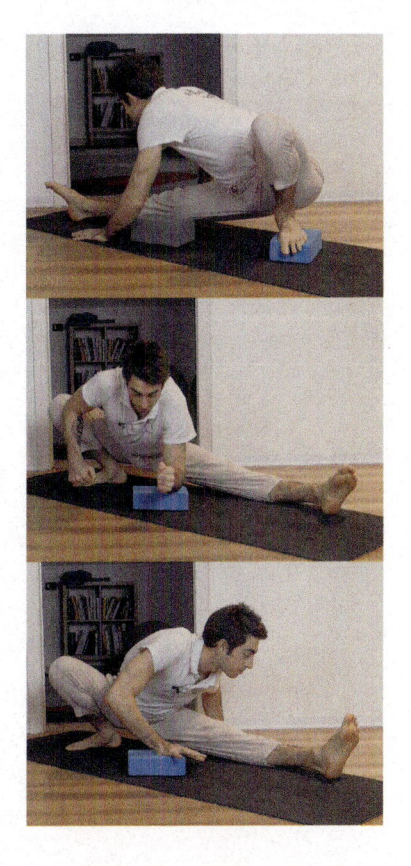

> Start in the **bottom** position of a **cossack squat**.
>
> Drive your **trunk down**, toward your straight leg, bent leg, or toward the center of your legs.

Part 3

—

SPECIFIC EXERCISES

SEATED GOOD MORNING

This is one of the best exercises you can use to develop your pancake position.

First of all, you want to start sitting on a bench, a chair, or similar support, then:

▸ **Spread your legs wide apart**. Squeeze your glutes to do that, and think about separating your knees.

▸ Make sure your **feet** stay exactly **below your knees**.

▸ Sit down with an **anterior pelvic tilt** activation. Drive your butt back and straighten your lower back.

At this point, you want to use a **weight**. You can either use a barbell or stick with some weights on it and put it behind your head, or take a dumbbell, kettlebell, or similar weight and hold it in front of your chest.

From the starting position, you want to drive your torso down as much as you can, keeping your back as straight as possible and pushing your knees constantly out. This will create a strong sensation of stretch on your adductors and hip extensors.

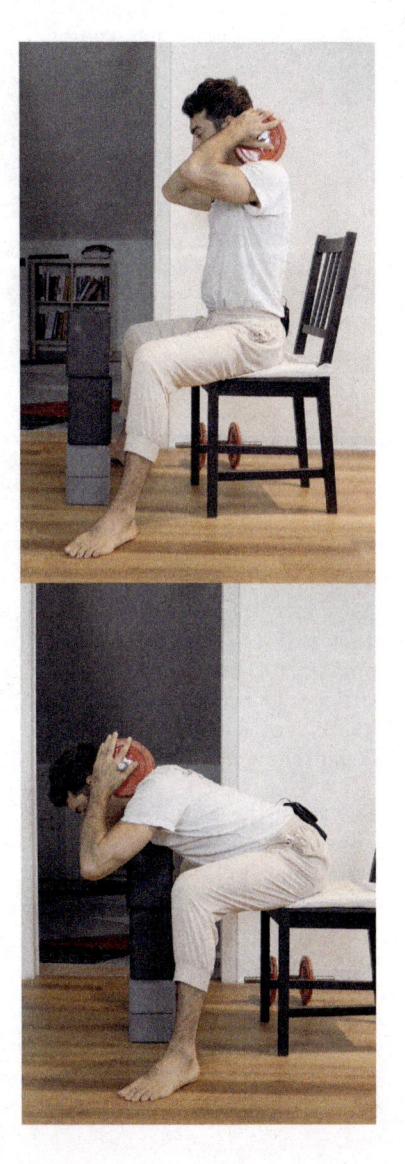

You want to **control** the way down as much as you can: make sure that the weight you're using is not too much and that you can get into a deep stretching position with it.

Once in the bottom position, stop there for a couple of seconds or more, driving your knees strongly out and your head in front of you; feel the stretch there, and come back up.

You can put some yoga blocks on top of the bench or on the floor (in case you're not using a bench) to keep track of your progress and measure how far you're going into the stretch.

As you get better and better, your goal is to bring your **torso parallel to the floor** without curving your lower and middle back too much and/or collapsing with your knees in.

Beware that these two types of compensations are really common and something you have to pay attention to: remember to push your knees out at all times and do your best to maintain your lower back straight, even though, in all honesty, it may curve a little: that's fine, don't be too scrupulous about that.

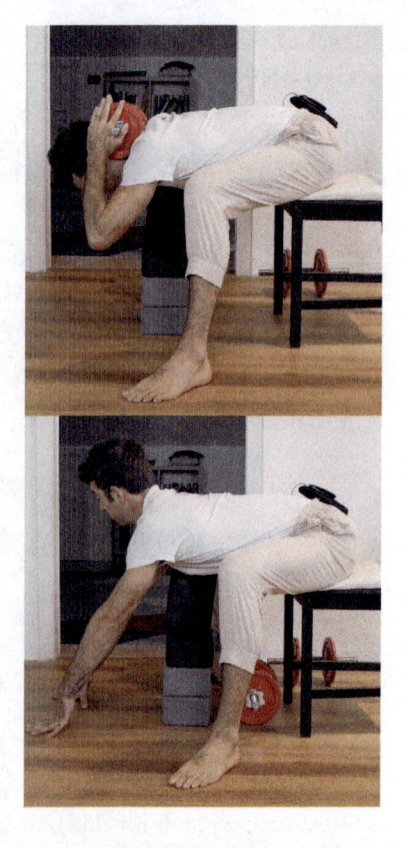

> Start in a seated position on a bench or a chair.
>
> Drive your **knee** strongly **out** and keep your lower back straight.
>
> Drive your **body down** using a **weight**.

74

HALF PANCAKE

The half pancake is an excellent exercise to work on your **hip internal rotation** and **hip abduction**, two important components of a good pancake. Plus, as the name suggests, it's a "half" pancake, meaning that your legs and hips are placed similarly to a pancake position.

Start sitting on the floor and spread your legs apart, forming approximately a 90° angle between them. Bend one leg and drive the foot of that leg behind your butt. Make sure to *point that toe* and relax your ankle, as I'm showing in the pictures on this page. If you do it correctly, you shouldn't feel any tension in the inner part of your bent knee. If you do feel that tension, bring your legs closer to each other.

Relax the bent leg's hip and gently push it down towards the floor. According to your flexibility level and your hip joint's structure, you may have that hip far away from the floor or completely pressed against it.

If you can't flatten your bent leg's hip on the floor yet, put a pillow or yoga block under it and gently push it towards the floor and the pillow.

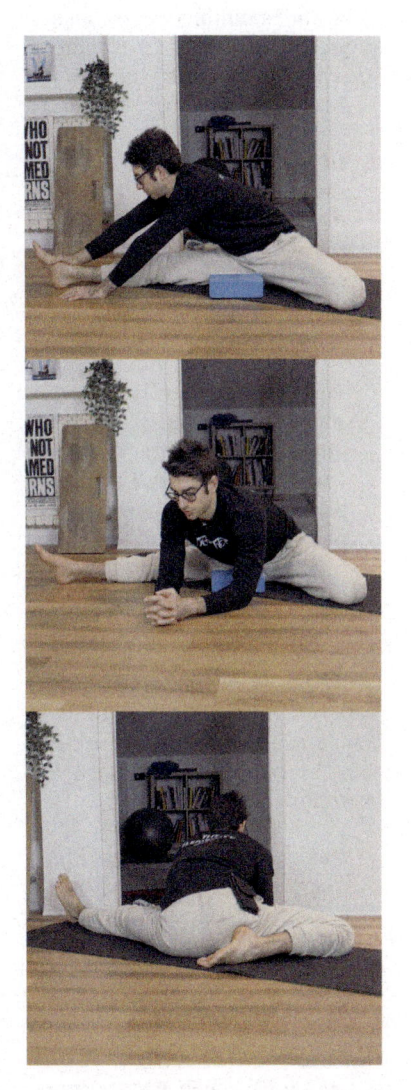

The other leg remains straight and externally rotated, with your foot pointing up. At this point, to create the *stretching effect*, you can drive your body in different directions:

▸ **In between the legs**. This is the most important one. Fold your trunk exactly in the middle of your legs. To do so, lean a little bit over the bent leg before going down into the stretch.

▸ **Towards the straight leg**. Turn your trunk in the direction of the straight leg, flatten the lower and middle back, keep the bent leg's hip pushed down and fold your trunk towards the straight leg.

Use some yoga blocks under your hands, elbows, or chest, depending on your flexibility level, to better relax into the stretch. To gain more range of motion, you can:

▸ **Pull towards something**. Place a weight on the floor or pull your body toward something.

▸ **PNF**. Push the straight leg's heel down against the floor. Hold the PNF contraction for 10 to 20", then gently stop, inhale, and on the exhale, try to get deeper into the stretch.

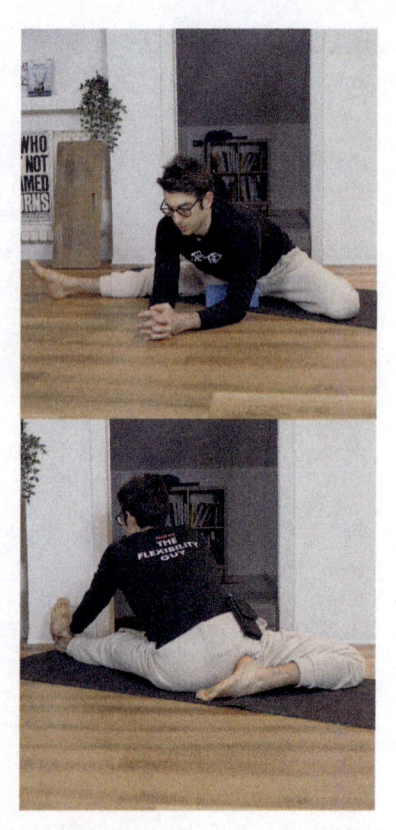

> Push your **bent leg's hip down**.
>
> You can drive your trunk in different directions.
>
> **PNF**: push your straight leg's heel against the floor.

RAISING FOOT PANCAKE STRETCH

Start in a standing position with a wall by your side. Place one foot on the wall slightly above your hips and press your hips toward the wall, keeping both legs straight.

Once in this position, which you can better see in the pictures on this page, you have two main options to **create** and/or **increase** the stretch.

▸ **Flex your trunk laterally** toward your leg.

▸ **Raise your foot up**, moving it higher on the wall.

Both strategies increase and create more stretch on your *hamstrings, your glutes, and your adductors* mostly.

You can use a **PNF contraction**, pushing your foot against the wall for 10 to 20", then stop, inhale, and on the exhale, try to get deeper using the strategies explained above, together or just one at a time.

How much you can raise your foot up depends on your flexibility level. The aim here is to raise your foot as much as you can until you can touch your trunk with your leg.

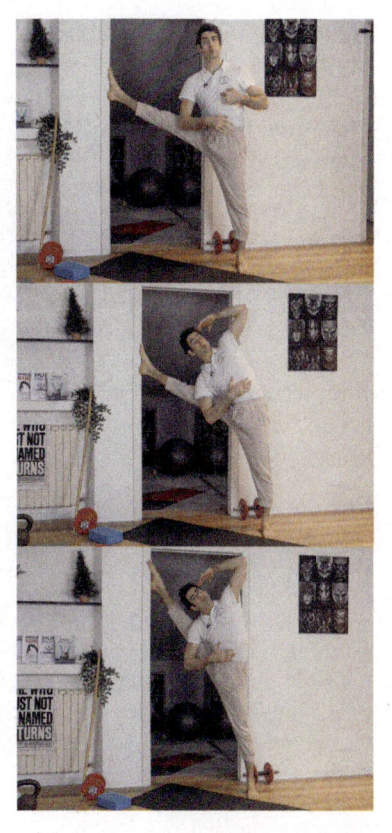

Keep both of your **legs straight**.

Raise your **foot up** or flex your **trunk laterally**.

PNF: push your foot against the wall.

77

STANDING PANCAKE STRETCH

This is one of the best pancake exercises you can do, as it has one huge advantage compared to the floor pancake. Rather than having your hips on the floor like in a classic pancake, your hips here are not on the floor. This gives them much more room to move, so you can better go into anterior pelvic tilt and fold your trunk toward the middle of your legs.

Start by standing on a support (like a bench) or two supports (like two chairs, etc.) with your legs opened, forming a 90° angle between them or a little more. **Use a weight** to pull yourself into the stretch, or **grab** the support **with your hands** and pull. Move your trunk toward your legs and your head down until you can feel the desired sensation of stretch. Remember to:

▶ **Anterior pelvic tilt**. Keep your lower back as straight as possible.

▶ Keep your legs **straight**.

You can perform a **dynamic** variation where you bend and extend both legs at the same time or one per time, or a **passive static** variation, where you stay in the stretch.

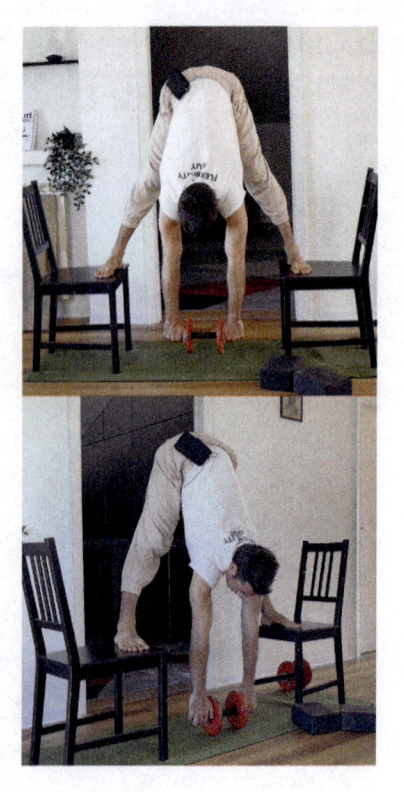

> Spread your **legs wide apart**.
>
> **Anterior pelvic tilt** and **straighten** your lower back.
>
> **Dynamic repetitions:** bend and extend your legs for reps.

BOX SPLIT

The box split is one of the best exercises you can use to develop **hip abduction** and **adductors** flexibility. I'm not going to lie to you: if you master the *splits*, the pancake will probably be a joke for you. That's why my first flexibility book has been *Splits Hacking*: with that kind of flexibility, your lower body really knows no limits (almost).

To perform a **box split**, start in a standing position, open your legs wide and put your hands on the floor, flexing your trunk forward.

Now the most important thing is to place something (I suggest yoga blocks) both **under your legs and under your chest** to relax on. This will create the right sensations of stretch and will be a good measure of your progress. Prioritize the position of the supports you have under your legs: once that is fixed, the supports under your chest will just follow that measure.

If you're a beginner, I suggest you place the supports *under your knees:* widen your legs, make sure your feet remain in line with your hips and touch the supports with your knees.

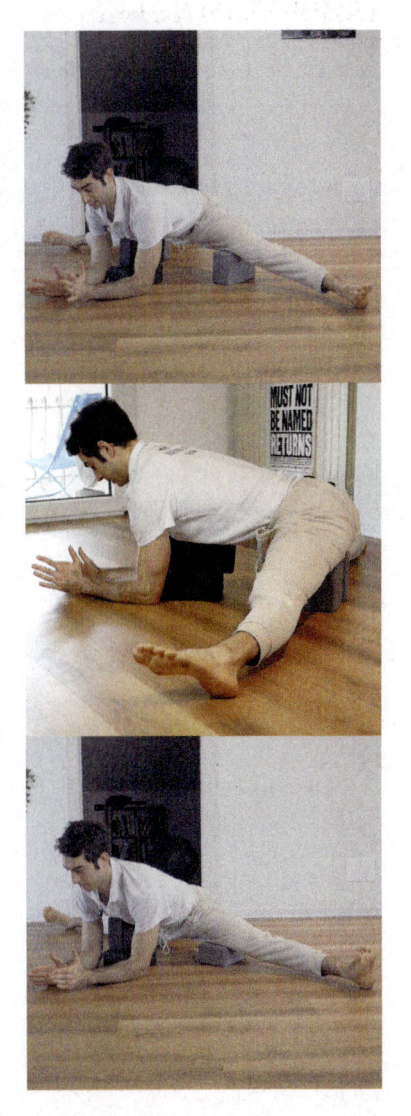

You can **adjust the height** of the supports, placing them in a *vertical or horizontal position* depending on the height you need. Once in that position, flex your body forward and put some supports under your chest.

There's a simple rule of thumb at this point: **you want to have your trunk almost parallel to the floor**, with your shoulders higher than your hips.

As you gain range of motion in the exercise, lower the supports and/or move them closer to your hips. Both strategies work well. A piece of advice I can give you here is to take it slow: **don't force the progression**. Move them when you're ready and little by little. Remember to:

- **Anterior pelvic tilt**.

- You can both **externally** or **internally** rotate your legs.
  If you externally rotate, your hamstrings will be stretched a little bit more, and vice versa; if you **internally rotate**, your adductors will be stretched a little more.

- Keep your feet, legs and hips on the same line.

To apply a **PNF contraction**, push your feet down. To apply an **antagonist contraction**, squeeze your glutes and push your feet up.

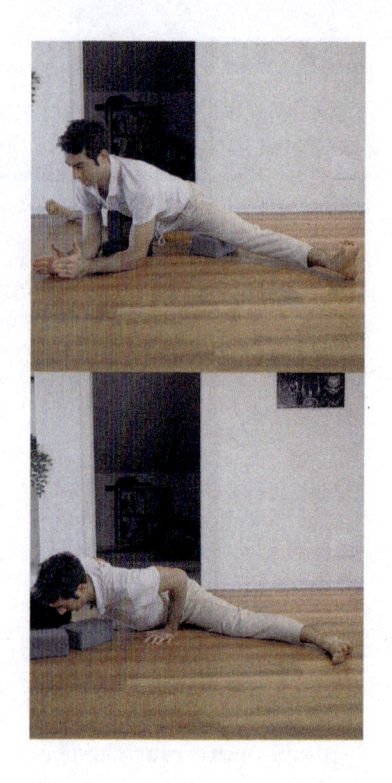

> Feet, legs and hips **on the same line**.
>
> Keep your **shoulders above your hips' level**.
>
> Put how many supports you need **under** your **legs** and your **chest**.

LATERAL PANCAKE

The lateral pancake is a side flexion movement where the trunk folds laterally towards one leg. This kind of stretch involves the *hip extensors,* the *adductors,* and, most importantly, a muscle you have deep inside your spine: the *quadratus lomborum*. This muscle, among the other functions, **extends the trunk and bends it laterally**. This means that if the *quadratus lomborum* is stiff, it prevents the forward bending motion typical of the pancake. That's why having it well stretched and flexible is a good idea to improve the pancake's range of motion.

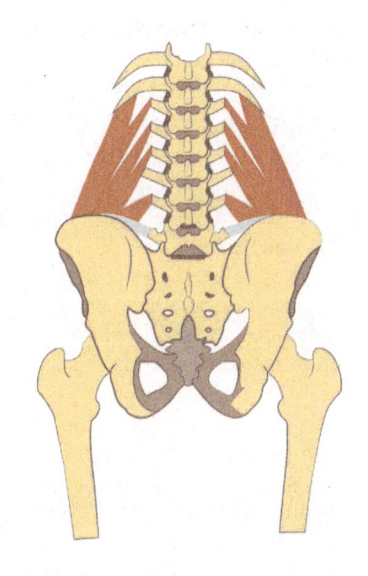

The quadratus lomborum.

We're going to see now some of the best progressions to work towards a complete lateral pancake stretch, starting from the easiest and ending with the final progression. The first one is the bent legs lateral pancake.

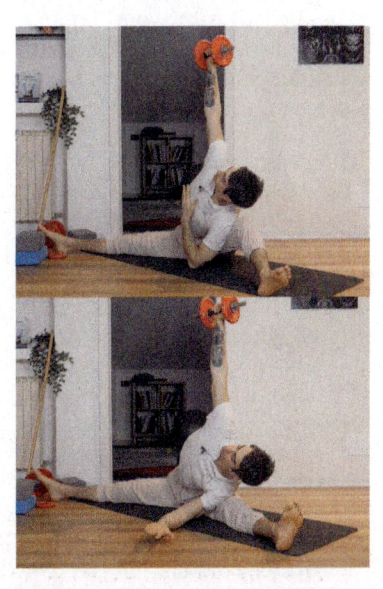

First of all, I'd like to make an important distinction between the two kinds of progressions we're going to use: the lateral pancake **on a bench** (or support) and the lateral pancake **on the floor**. You want to start with the one on the bench, which is easier, then move to the harder one on the floor.

LATERAL PANCAKE ON BENCH

Sit down at the edge of a bench with one leg on the bench and the other on the floor. If you don't have a bench, you can use a couple of chairs.

You want to keep the leg on the bench flexed at approximately 90 degrees to start. Fold your trunk **laterally** towards the leg you have on the bench, trying to keep it *as perpendicular to the floor as possible*. As you do so, **push your bottom shoulder forward** and your **top shoulder back:** this will help you keep your trunk in the correct position. You can grab the bench with your bottom hand and pull your bottom shoulder forward to make this happen.

Don't lift your opposite hip off the bench as you go into the stretch! Keep it well-pressed down. To gain more range of motion, use these strategies.

▸ **Weight on the top hand**. Grab a weight with your top hand and let it push your trunk down toward the leg. When you use a weight, you can perform a **dynamic stretch,** driving your trunk down and up, and a **static stretch**, letting the weight push your trunk down toward your leg.

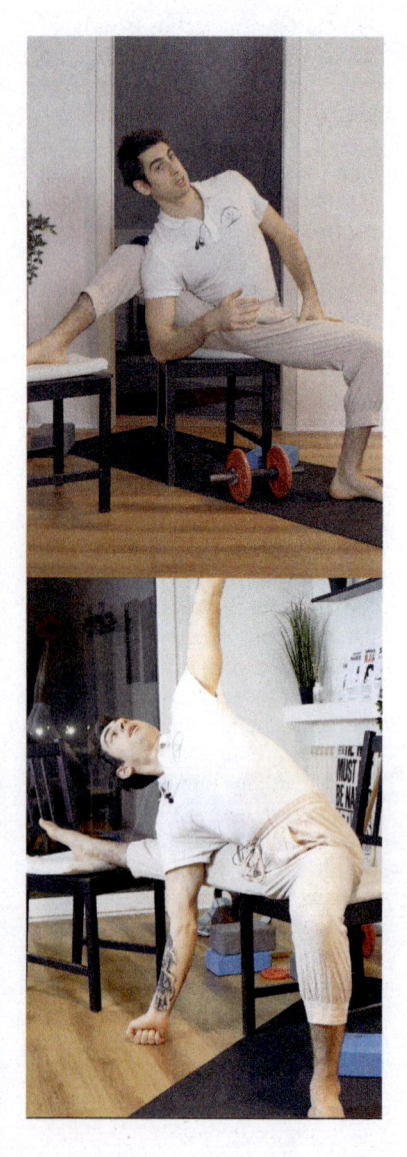

▸ **PNF**: push with the heel of your leg against the bench. Hold the contraction for 10 to 20", then stop, inhale, and on the exhale, get deeper into the stretch.

A good strategy I suggest you use during a lateral pancake is **putting a yoga block between your trunk and the leg** you're leaning on: in this way, you'll better relax into the stretch and keep track of your progress.

Once you can touch your leg with your trunk, you can progress by extending your leg more. This doesn't mean you have to **completely straighten** your leg: it does mean that you want to **progressively get there** by extending your leg little by little: every time you can touch your trunk with your leg, try to straighten it a little more.

You can also directly try the **straight leg** lateral pancake on the bench; in this case, as I said, I suggest you put something between your leg and your trunk to better relax into the stretch. This straight leg variation is surely harder as it requires *more hamstrings flexibility*, so pay extra attention to the position of your opposite hip: don't lift it off the bench as you flex your body laterally.

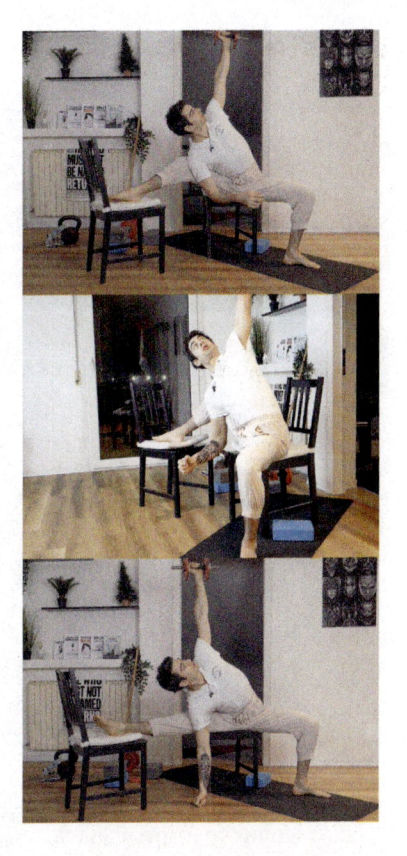

One leg on a bench.

Flex your trunk laterally toward your leg, keeping it bent or straight.

Use a **weight** to get deeper into the stretch.

LATERAL PANCAKE

The progression you want to follow for a lateral pancake is completely identical to the one explained for the bench lateral pancake: you want to first start with your leg bent, gently leaning over it, keeping your trunk as perpendicular to the floor as possible. Then you want to **gradually extend** your leg until it is straight.

This time, though, you're going to perform this exercise on the floor, which makes the task a little harder. Start with both of your hips on the floor in a seated position and your legs straight. Now bend one leg, and lean toward that side. You want to use your bottom hand to grab your opposite foot and pull your bottom shoulder forward as you gently flex the torso laterally: in this way, you're going to experiment a much deeper and more intense stretch, as your trunk will be forced to stay as perpendicular to the floor. If you can't reach the foot, wrap a band around it.

Pay particular attention to this really common mistake: you **don't lift your hips off the floor** as you move your trunk. Both of your glutes must be well-pressed against the floor at all times, especially the one on your opposite side.

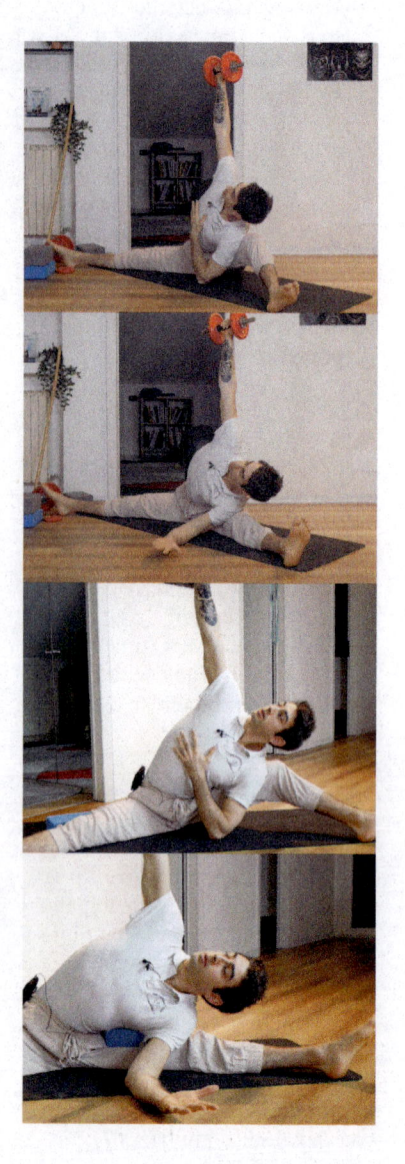

You can use **two strategies** to get into the stretch.

- **Weight on the top hand**. Grab a weight with your top hand and let it push your trunk down toward the leg. When you use a weight, you can perform a **dynamic stretch,** driving your trunk down and up, and a **static stretch**, letting the weight push your trunk down toward your leg.

- **PNF**: push with the heel of your leg against the floor. Hold the contraction for 10 to 20", then stop, inhale, and on the exhale, get deeper into the stretch.

When you can touch your leg with your trunk, you can extend your leg more, and if you can't yet, **put a yoga block between your trunk and the leg** to better relax into the stretch.

The fact that you want to make progress when you can touch your leg with your trunk doesn't mean you can't perform the **straight leg variation**. I'm telling you this just to give you a sense of progression, but of course, you can work on both the **bent** and **straight** leg variations whenever you want; just make sure to follow the correct technique.

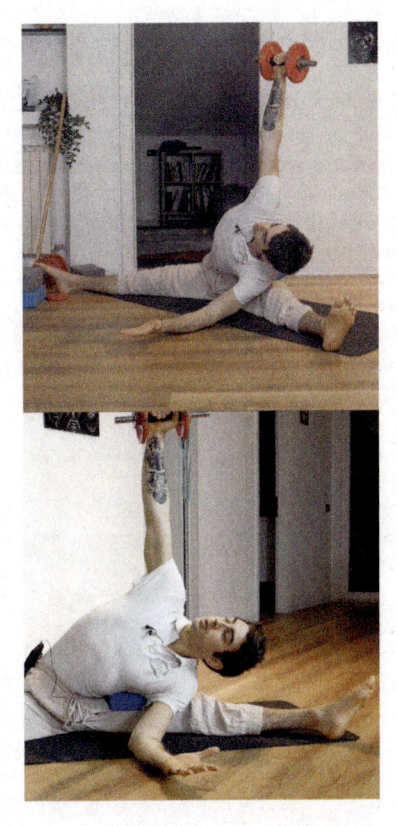

> Seated on the floor, both of your legs straight.
>
> **Flex your trunk laterally** toward one leg, keeping it bent or straight.
>
> Use a **weight** to get deeper into the stretch.

BENT LEGS AND STRAIGHT LEGS PANCAKE

There are two major distinctions we're going to make for the pancake stretch. You can do a pancake stretch with your legs **straight** or **bent**, and you can do a pancake with your **butt elevated** or **on the floor.**

First, we're going to explore the different techniques you can use (listed above), then we're going to see the best range of motion strategies you can use to create a high number of combinations you can use in your training to increase your flexibility level.

Now, let's see the first *two variations*: **bent legs** and **straight legs** pancakes.

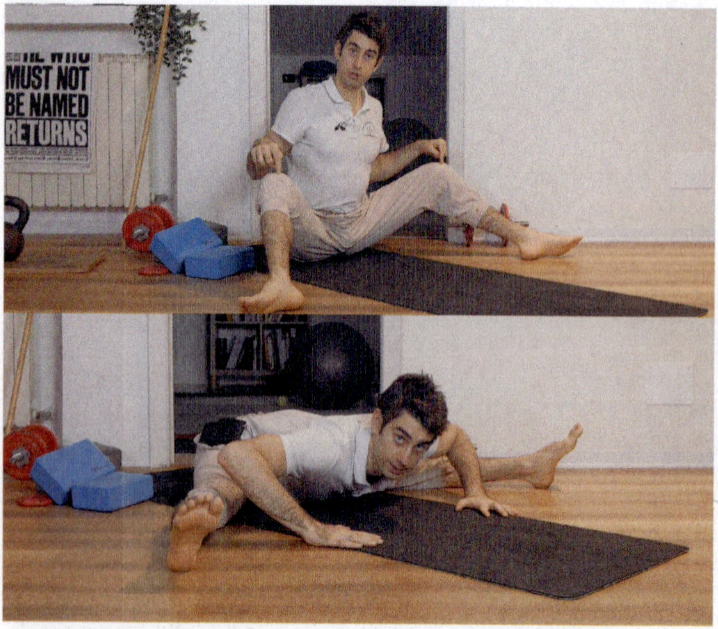

Figure 13. Bent legs and straight legs pancakes.

BENT LEGS PANCAKE

You may wonder why you should bend your knees at this point. The reason is that this will put a little less stretch on your hamstrings (*only the portion closer to your knees*) and your calves, allowing you to focus the stretch more on your adductors and the upper portion of your hamstrings. This is critical to developing a better hip position in a pancake stretch. Bending your knees also makes it easier to **externally rotate** your legs: just think about driving your knees back, and your legs will externally rotate by a good measure.

How much should you bend the knees? I suggest from **30° to 70°** of knee flexion. Play with those angles and find the one where you can feel your adductors and hamstrings in the best stretch possible.

A very important note: it will be hard, much harder compared to the classic variation of a pancake, to touch your chest and belly with the floor during a bent legs pancake. This is not the purpose of this stretch. The aim here is to aim for the max range of motion possible: place some supports under your chest to relax on and keep track of your progress.

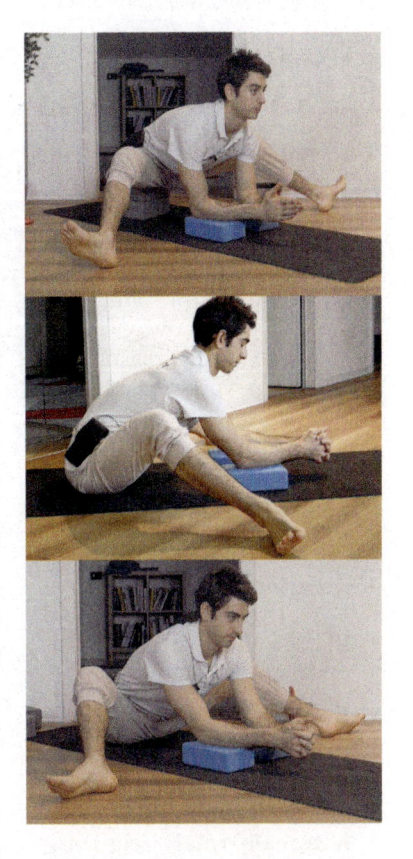

Bent legs, 30°/70° of knee flexion.

Externally rotate your legs.

All the other pancake technique rules remain exactly the same.

STRAIGHT LEGS PANCAKE

The straight legs pancake is the "*classic*" variation of the pancake, nothing special to say about it since we covered all the details of the pancake in the introduction section. Despite that, it is always good to point out another time all the major things you need to care about during a *straight legs pancake* position.

▸ Keep your **legs** completely **straight**.

▸ **Anterior pelvic tilt**.

▸ Flatten your lower and middle back as much as you can.

▸ Open your chest, and push your head forward.

▸ **Externally rotate** your legs. It will be harder compared to the bent legs variation. Push your toes back and point your knees up.

▸ Drive your trunk in between your legs.

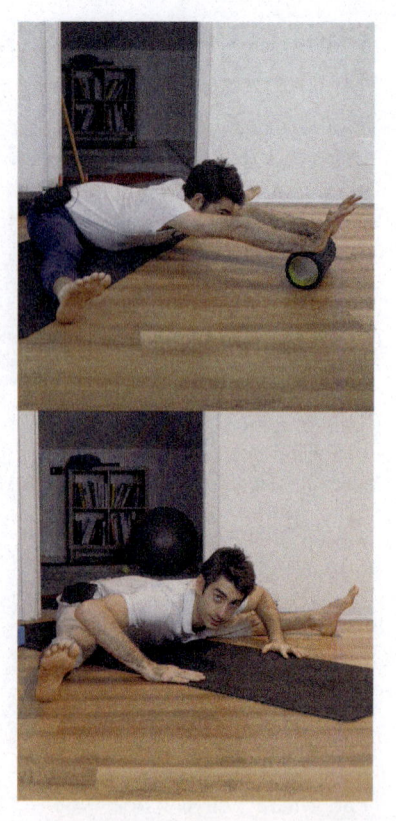

> Keep your **legs** completely **straight**.
>
> **Externally rotate** your legs.

BUTT ELEVATED AND PANCAKE ON THE FLOOR

Let's talk about this very important technique you can use to reach your pancake stretch, which is, in my opinion, one of the best ones you can use to **increase your flexibility**.

As for the previous variations, one is the "strange", the "unusual", and "unknown", while the other one is the "standard" one that most people know. Please take note that both the *bent and straight legs* pancake can be done with the **butt elevated** or on **the floor**.

I'm not going to talk about the floor pancake, as it respects the same rules and activations we've been seeing so far for the standard pancake.

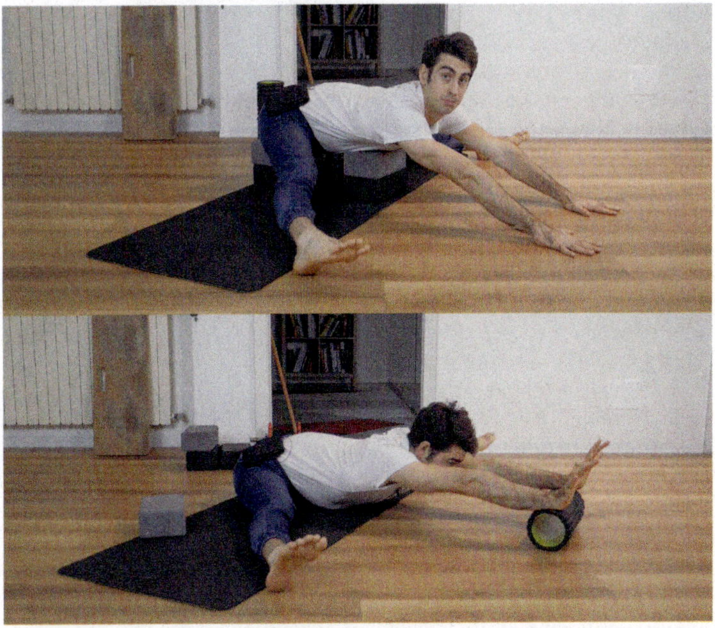

Figure 14. Butt elevated and pancake on the floor.

BUTT-ELEVATED PANCAKE

We're going to see now what, for me, is the most important progression to reach the pancake stretch.
As I previously said, this strategy can be used in each and every specific pancake position you can think of.

The starting position is exactly the one you use in a pancake. This time, though, you don't want to sit on the floor, but you want to put some **supports under your hips**. This will incline your legs and, depending on the **height** you use, make the exercise *easier*: the higher the supports, the easier the exercise, and vice versa. The exercise gets easier because when you raise your hips up, you decrease the stretch on them.

Even though you may not notice, when you sit down on the floor with your legs straight, your hamstrings and glutes go under stretch. As a matter of fact, a lot of people struggle just to sit down on the floor with their legs straight, as their hamstrings and glutes pull so strongly that they can't properly sit. The stiffer your hamstrings, the less you can stay in a seated position with your legs straight.

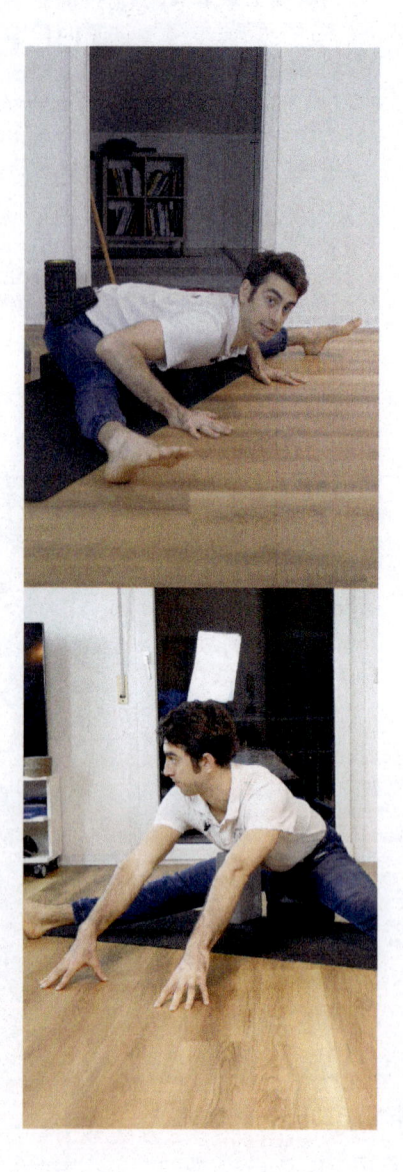

90

When you move your hips up, things change, though: the stretch on your hips **decreases** as the angle between your legs and your trunk becomes less and less demanding.

At this point, once you're well positioned, you can use all the pancake range of motion techniques we're going to see in the next few pages, but make sure to follow the following progression to get better.

▸ **Set the height** of the supports you want to keep under your hips. I usually suggest no more than your knees' height.

▸ Sit down on the supports, spread your legs wide apart, and **fold your trunk in between your legs**. Here I'm not going to get specific about the progressions you want to use, but since you want to perform a pancake, I can assume your trunk has to go toward your legs.

▸ As you fold your trunk down, you want to use some **yoga blocks** or another kind of support **under your chest**. This is critical as it measures the depth of the position and how deep you can go into the stretch.

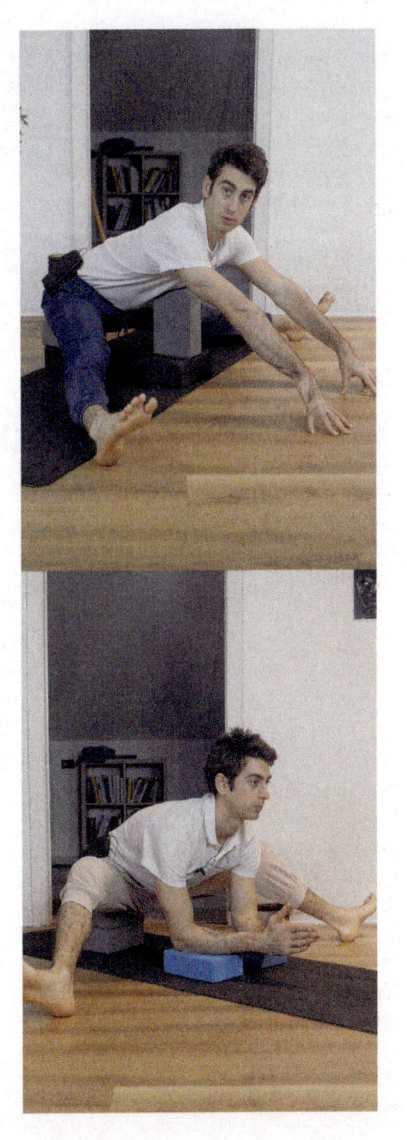

▶ **Here comes the important part.** You want to fold your trunk down and touch something with your chest, doesn't matter how high. As you make progress, move that something under your chest down **until it's at the same height** as the supports you have under your hips. At that point, your trunk will be **parallel** to the floor.

Once you have your trunk parallel to the floor, it is time for you to **make progress**: lower the supports under your hips and perform the butt-elevated pancake stretch from a different height, which is going to make the exercise harder.

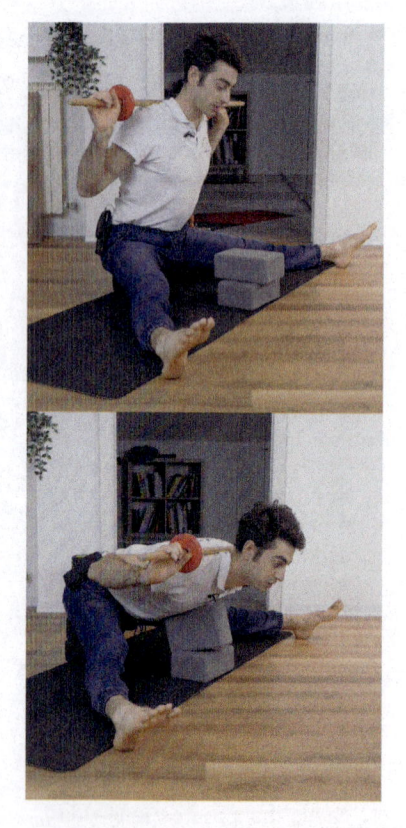

Sit down on some **yoga blocks** or another kind of support.

Bring your torso **parallel to the floor** in order to make progress.

PANCAKE RANGE OF MOTION TECHNIQUES

Let's make a little recap of all the different pancake variations we've seen.

- **Bent** legs pancake.
- **Straight** legs pancake.
- **Butt-elevated** pancake.
- **Floor** pancake.

These are the different techniques you can use during a pancake stretch. What we want to explore now are the **strategies** you can use to gain range of motion, no matter the pancake technique you're using. These strategies can be done in each and every pancake technique we've seen so far; you just have to combine them.

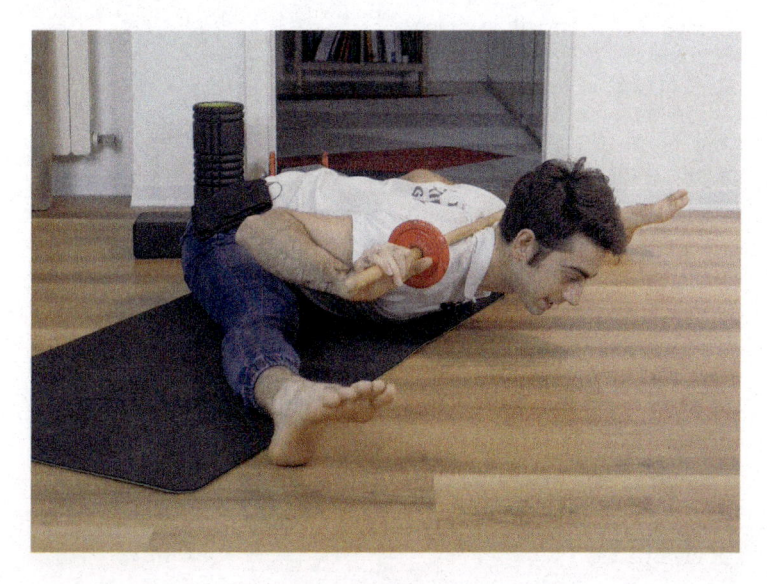

Figure 15. Weighted pancake.

PANCAKE EXTENSION

The pancake extension is a beautiful progression you can use to achieve the pancake stretch, and it uses the same principle we've seen for the seated good morning, only this time, you have to keep your legs straight and stay in a pancake position (remember this works in a bent legs, straight legs, butt-elevated and/or floor pancake).

Start in a pancake position and put a weight on your back. It can be a barbell, a dumbbell, or a stick with some weights on it. Open your chest, straighten your back, and move your hips into anterior pelvic tilt as much as possible. The sensation you want to feel is that you're not sitting on your glutes but on your *hip bones*, the bones you have at the bottom of your pelvis.

Put some yoga blocks in front of you. Drive your trunk down in between your legs until you can touch the yoga blocks with your chest, pause for a couple of seconds there, and come back up. Repeat for reps, usually 6 to 10, and on the final one, remain in the bottom position a little longer, like 5 to 10 breaths.

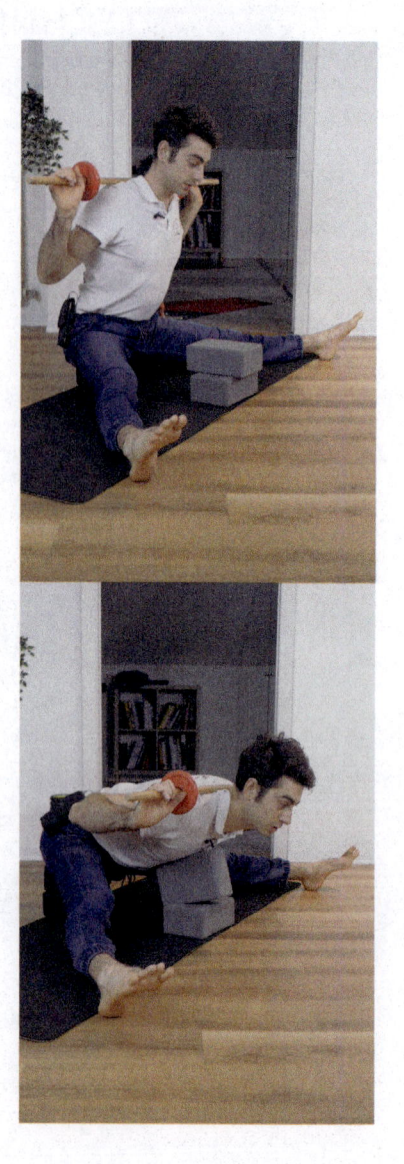

It is important for you to understand now the difference between the two positions you can maintain at the bottom of each rep because it changes a lot the stretch you're going to feel.

▸ You can drive your trunk down and, once in the bottom position, **hold the position with the strength of your muscles**. Here you don't want to relax on the yoga blocks: as a matter of fact, you barely want to touch them. They're there just to let you know how far you're going into the stretch, no more than that.

▸ You can drive your trunk down and **relax on the yoga blocks**. In this case, you're not using your muscles to stay in the stretching position: you're letting the weight push your trunk down and against the yoga blocks, and you're totally relaxing there.

Both of these strategies use a **loaded stretch**, but in the first case, you hold the position with the strength of your muscles in the bottom part. In the second case, instead, you use the assistance of the weight to better relax into the stretch. I suggest you mix both of these strategies for the best results.

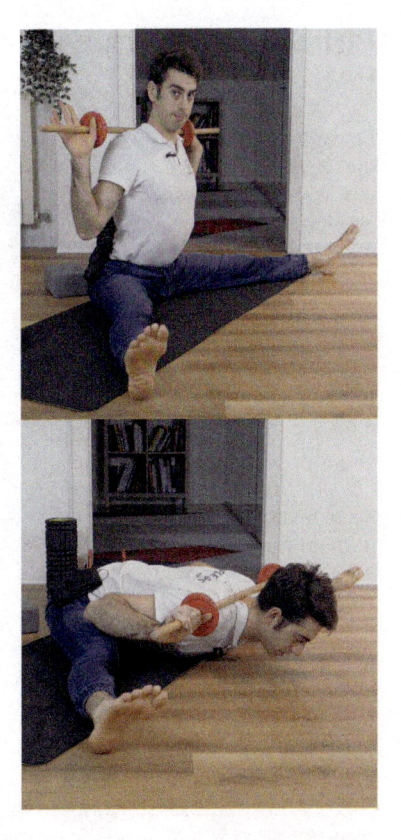

Butt-elevated to start, then on the floor.

Use a weight and move your trunk in between your legs.

Keep your back and legs straight at all times.

PULLING INTO A PANCAKE

During a pancake extension, the exercise we've just seen, you want to use a weight to get deeper and deeper into a stretching position, right? Well, here, you want to use the exact same kind of reasoning, but rather than using a weight, you want to use the strength of your arms to pull yourself deeper and deeper into the stretch.

As a matter of fact, in order to perform this exercise, you have to have something in front of you to **pull yourself toward**, like a support, a weight, a stall bar, a piece of furniture, or a chair with some weights on it... Something stable that won't move.

Now, you want to start in a pancake stretch with your legs wide apart. You can put some yoga blocks under your hips or not; this is your choice: the exercise works the same for both variations. Same for keeping your legs straight or bent. Fold your trunk in between your legs, reach out with your hands, and grab the support in front of you. At this point, pull yourself into the stretch strongly, trying to compress your torso toward your legs as much as possible.

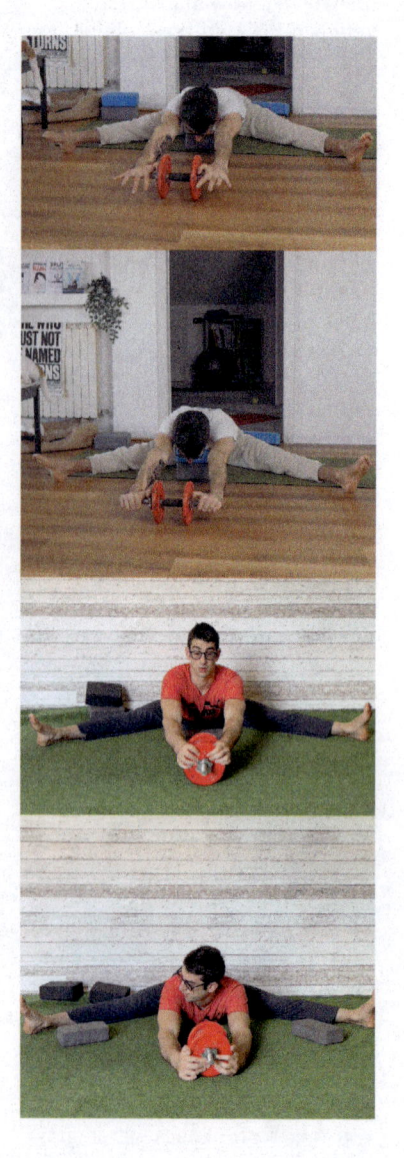

As you reach the bottom position, stop there and try to straighten your back as much as possible, pushing your head in front of you. You can use a couple of strategies to gain more range of motion.

- **PNF**. Push your feet against the floor for a count of 10 to 20", then stop, inhale, and on the exhale, get deeper into the stretch.

- Every couple of breaths, pull yourself **deeper** into the stretch.

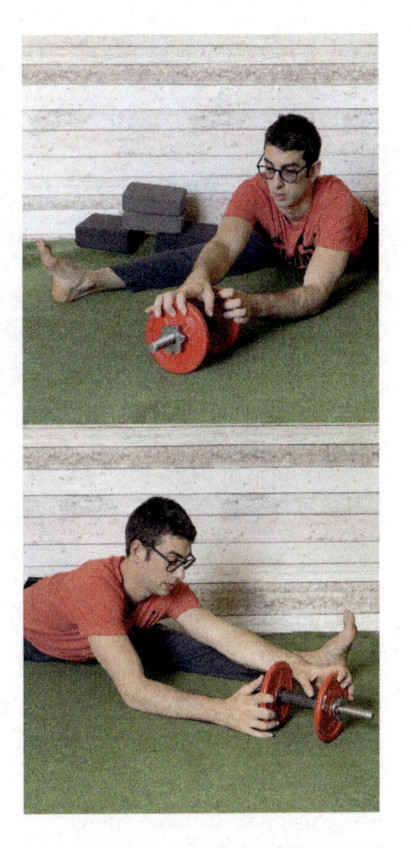

> **Butt-elevated** to start, then on the floor.
>
> **Pull** yourself deeper and deeper into the stretch using your arms' strength
>
> **PNF**: push your heels against the floor.

ROLLING INTO PANCAKE

This is a really simple strategy you can use to gain more range of motion, as it's an excellent dynamic stretch for your pancake. Not the strongest one, but I do think it does its job pretty well.

Start in a pancake position with your torso upright and your hands on a foam roller, ab wheel or slippery surface. From there, fold your trunk down in between the legs keeping your hands on the foam roller, which will roll forward and pull your hands deeper and deeper into the stretch. Once in the deepest stretch possible, stay there for a brief moment there, then roll back into the starting position.

Since this is a dynamic stretch, you'll feel that rep after rep, your range of motion increases up until a certain point, of course. I suggest you perform 6 to 10 dynamic and controlled repetitions, and on the last one, remain in the stretch for the last 5 to 10 breaths.

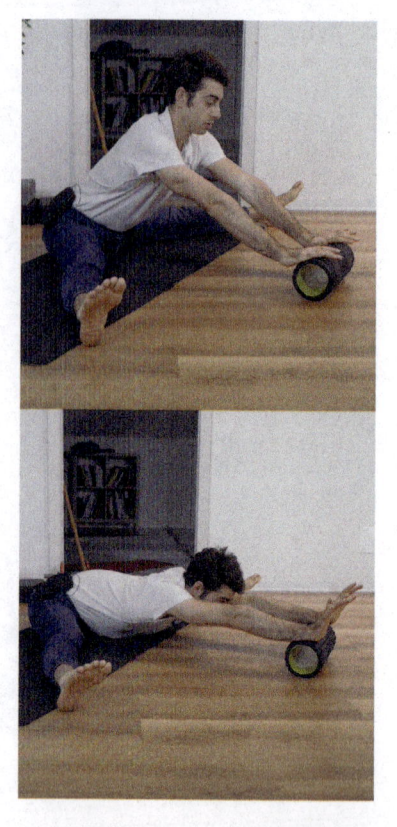

Roll your trunk down letting your arms slide **in front and away** from you.

Increase your range of motion rep by rep.

PANCAKE WALKS

The principle that stays behind a pancake walk is that by moving your trunk in **different directions** during a pancake, you're going to stretch your muscles from different angles, gaining flexibility where you need it the most. Let's assume, for instance, that your left leg is **stiffer** than your right. During a pancake walk, you want to move your body toward your left leg, which as a consequence of that, is going to be stretched more since this lateral movement is going to focus the stretch on that leg, something that wouldn't have happened if you only practiced the regular variation.

So, start in a pancake stretch, move your body toward your right leg, and grab your foot or your ankle with your hands. Pull yourself into the stretch. From there, slowly move your trunk toward your left, pushing it as close to the floor as possible, then a little more, and a little more again... Take **small steps** toward the center until you're exactly in the middle of your legs. Now little steps toward the left, pausing in each position you find for a couple of seconds (or more, if you feel particularly stiff there). That's one rep. You can repeat the whole process for 4 to 6 reps.

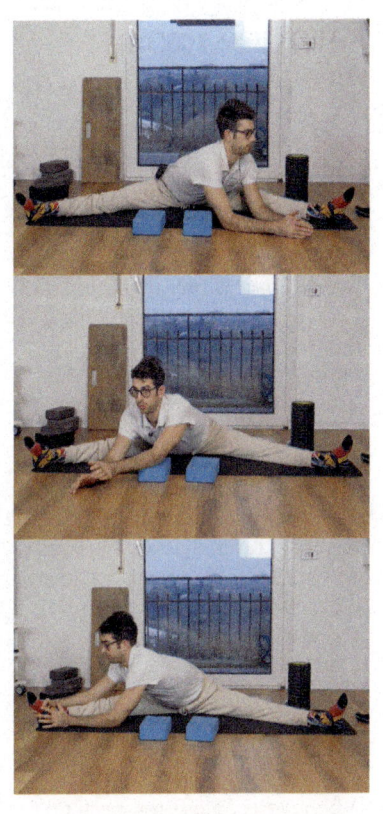

Start in a pancake position, and move your body toward your **right and left leg**.

Keep pushing your trunk down at all times.

Keep your back and legs straight at all times.

PARTNER-ASSISTED PANCAKE

I still remember the first time I managed to do a flat pancake on the floor. I was in my gym, and I was trying to get into the deepest pancake stretch I could. Only a few centimeters were separating my chest and abdominals from the floor, but damn, those centimeters were feeling like kilometers!

Frustrated, I asked my girlfriend to sit down gently on my lower back in order to push my body further down. She sat slowly, letting me absorb the additional weight little by little. My trunk slowly got into a deeper and deeper pancake stretch until I finally touched the floor with my chest and abdominals.

When it comes to partner-assisted stretching, I have no doubts: this is one of the best stretching methodologies you can use to increase your flexibility and range of motion. Unfortunately, not everyone has access to a stretching partner who can help her stretch and get deeper into the positions. This is why in my books, I rarely propose partner-assisted exercises and prefer stretches that everyone can do with minimal equipment.

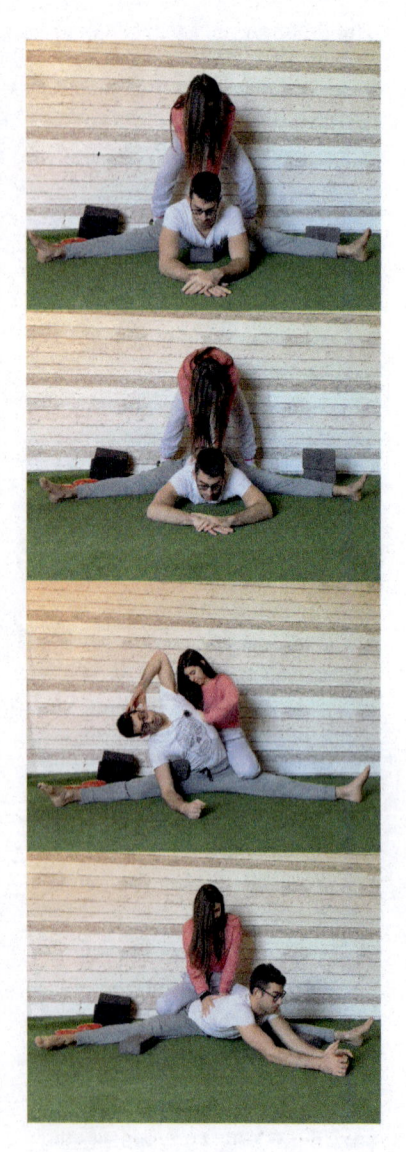

This time, though, I'd like to make a little exception. A partner-assisted pancake is surely a golden exercise you can use to achieve your flat pancake stretch. If you stretch with someone else, you have a gym-bro, a son or a daughter who're in your proximities when you stretch, or whomever you want, give this strategy a go.

You can use whatever kind of pancake technique you want, bent legs, butt-elevated, straight legs... Your choice! When you are in the stretching position, ask your partner to **gently** push your trunk down and in whichever direction you prefer. If, for example, you want to perform the pancake walks, you can ask the partner to push your body a little more toward your left, your right, etc.

The communication between you and your partner is **critical**. You must always be in control of the stretch, not your partner. Ask him or her to provide the amount of assistance **you need**, feel right for your flexibility level, and find the intensity you want.

Your partner can push you down into the stretch by pushing with her or his hands, or as in my story, sit down on your back. Keyword: **gently**.

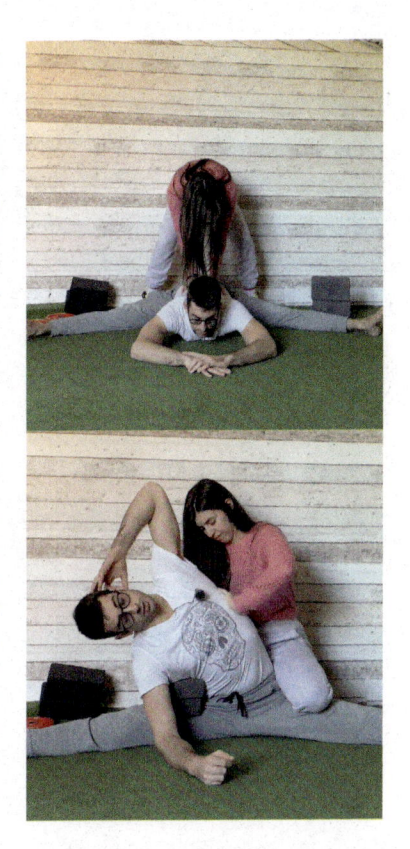

> Use the assistance of a partner to get **deeper** and deeper into a pancake position.
>
> The assistance must be **gradual**, **gentle**, and not too intense.

PASSIVE PANCAKE

This one is the version I like the less. Staying "only" passively in a pancake position, without any kind of assistance, surely **is not** the best way to **develop** it since you can't adjust the intensity of the stretch as you want, which is something critical and that you can do with all the strategies listed above. I see the **passive** pancake only as a *final result*: once you've built a good flexibility level, you want to test it out by staying passively in the pancake stretch without any external force to help.

That being said, the passive pancake is the hardest position to reach, though: nothing can help you here! Not a weight, not your arms, not a partner. Nothing. You must activate your body correctly and get into a flat pancake with passive flexibility only.

- Anterior pelvic tilt.

- Externally rotate your legs.

- Flatten your lower and middle back. Drive your head forward to emphasize this.

- You can apply a PNF contraction by pushing both of your heels against the floor.

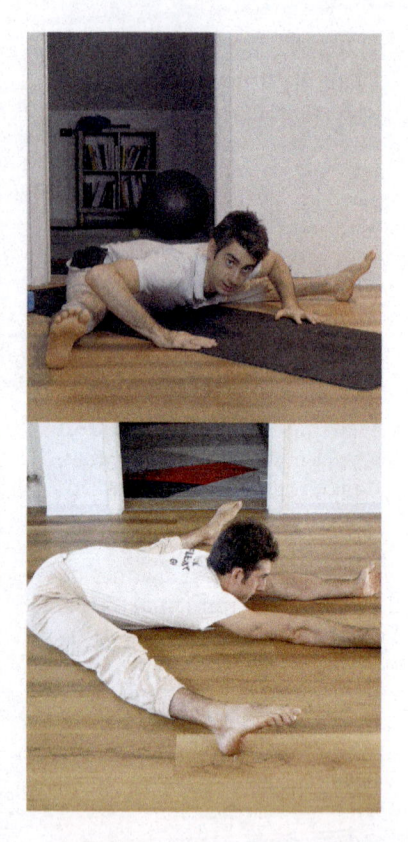

> Not so good to develop the pancake, this is more a **test** to see where you're at.
>
> **PNF**: push your heels against the floor.

OVER-PANCAKE

If you want to further increase your pancake stretch and forward bending range of motion, you can consider the **over-pancake**. In a standard pancake, you have your torso in line with your legs since both rests on the floor. You want to go beyond this in an over-pancake, bringing your trunk past your legs' level.

Some people do an over-pancake with one or more blocks under their feet, and even though that's accepted as the "common" way to do it, I think this is **wrong and bad for your knees**. Let me tell you why. In my opinion, raising only the feet off the floor and keeping all the other structures in the same place during a pancake position will over-stretch the knee joint.

As a matter of fact, it's really common to see people in an "over-pancake" with their heels on the supports and their knees touching the floor. If we analyzed the angle between legs and trunk in people performing the over-pancake with such a technique, we'd clearly see how it doesn't change from a regular pancake: the only thing that changes is the hyperextension of the knees.

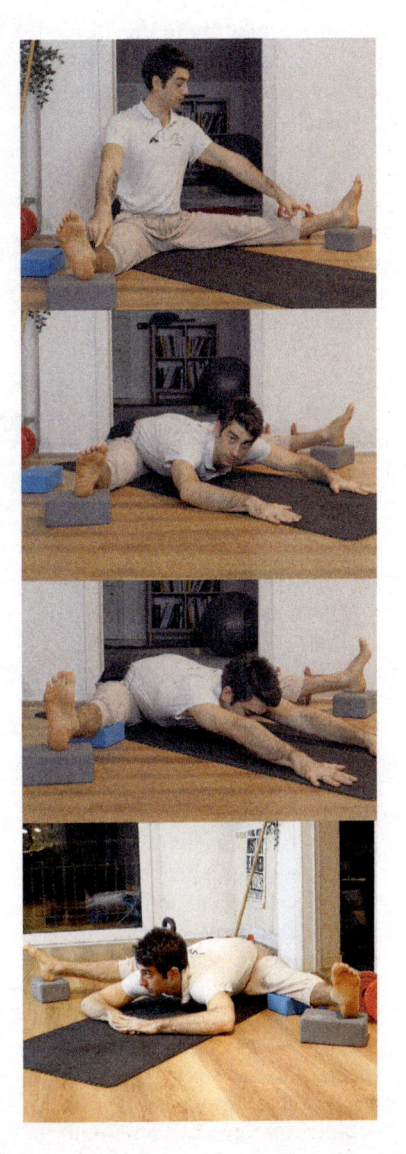

Hyperextension, though, can be very dangerous and produce severe instability in the knee cap. Moreover, the range won't come from the hips (where it should be) but from the knees!

With all these problems laid out, I'd like to show you now my personal view on this exercise with what, for me, is an intelligent "*solution*" to the hyperextension problem.

The solution is simple: you want to put some yoga blocks **under your feet and your knees**. In this way, there will be little to no hyperextension in the knees, and you'll be forced to gain range of motion through the hips, which is what you want to improve in a pancake!

That said, the **over-pancake technique** stays the same as for a regular pancake: anterior pelvic tilt, flatten your lower back, externally rotate your legs and drive your tummy down. You can use all the **strategies** we've been seeing so far to gain range of motion: weights, PNF, rolling, pulling, etc.

Always remember to put some blocks under your chest to better relax into the stretch and keep track of your progress.

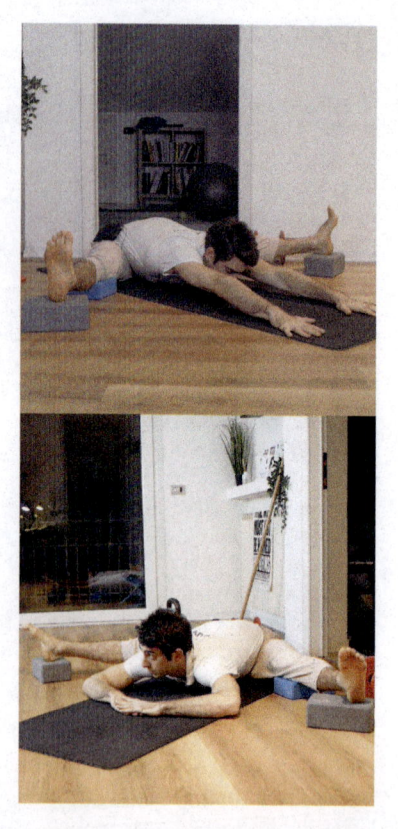

Put the yoga blocks both under your feet **and** your knees.

Fold your trunk down following the correct pancake technique.

LYING PANCAKE STRETCH

The lying pancake is maybe the "ultimate" pancake position, as in this stretch, you're not able to compensate with your back: you have to keep it super-straight at all times.

Start lying on your back with your glutes and lower back **well-pressed against the floor**. Straighten your legs, open them wide apart, grab your feet with your hands and pull them down toward the floor. You can wrap some weights around your feet to get deeper into the stretch. Bring your legs towards your chest, trying to mimic a pancake position, as shown in the pictures on this page.

You don't want to move your hips as you move your legs down. You want to constantly push them down toward the floor as you bring your legs toward your torso.

Even though this is not one of the strongest stretches we've seen, I do think it's an excellent test you can use to understand **how's your pancake flexibility**: if you can keep your entire back on the floor and touch the floor with your feet, you've surely **mastered the pancake** position.

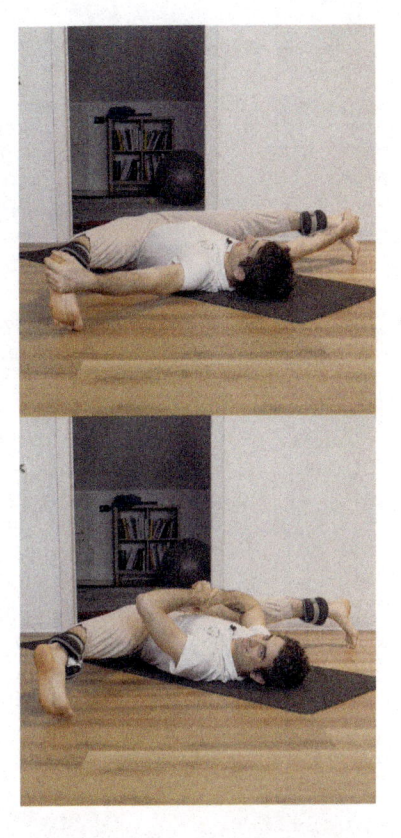

Lie down with your back on the floor.

Keep your legs straight and pull them toward your chest.

The **ultimate pancake flexibility test.**

A FINAL NOTE ON TECHNIQUE

I'd like to spend a couple of words now on the "correct technique" for a pancake. I always suggest not being fooled by the *"perfect form"*: perfection is something you pursue every day, little by little, and the pancake is for sure not an exception.

Your first aim should be touching the floor with your chest at first. It doesn't matter if you're a little bit curved with the lower and middle back: it's impossible to get a *"perfect"* pancake without going through the intermediate steps, and curving a little bit your lower and middle back is part of being intermediate. I see a lot of people just stopping far away from the floor in a pancake because they're *afraid* of getting deeper because their backs would curve after a certain point. That doesn't make any sense! Curving your back a bit is totally fine, especially when you're mastering the position.

There is a huge difference between doing your best to keep your back as straight as possible and maybe having it a little curved and curving the back on purpose without any kind of thought about straightening it. You want to be in the first category. After you can touch your chest to the floor, go for belly to the floor. After belly to the floor, think about a perfectly flat lower and middle back. That's the last stage, and it's something people reach after months or years of practice.

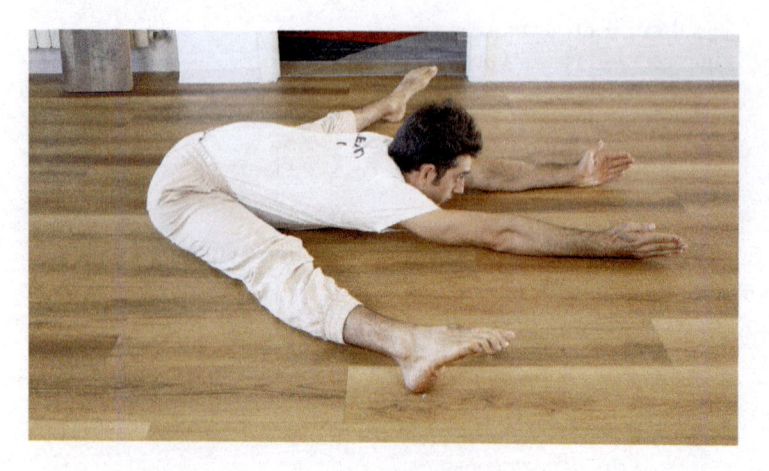

Figure 16. The pancake position.

Part 4

WORKOUT DESIGN

WORKOUT DESIGN

Now you have all the information and all the exercises in order to reach a correct pancake stretch.

The question is: what's going to lead you from theory to results? **Practice**. You should know how to practice and, more specifically, design a good workout program for the best results you can get.

I will provide you with three main examples of programs, starting from beginner, then intermediate, and advanced. Each program is designed in a certain way, and the thing I'd like to focus on the most is the logic behind the program, not the program itself. Once you understand the logic behind each program, you'll be perfectly able to personalize it to you, following your own needs and preferences.

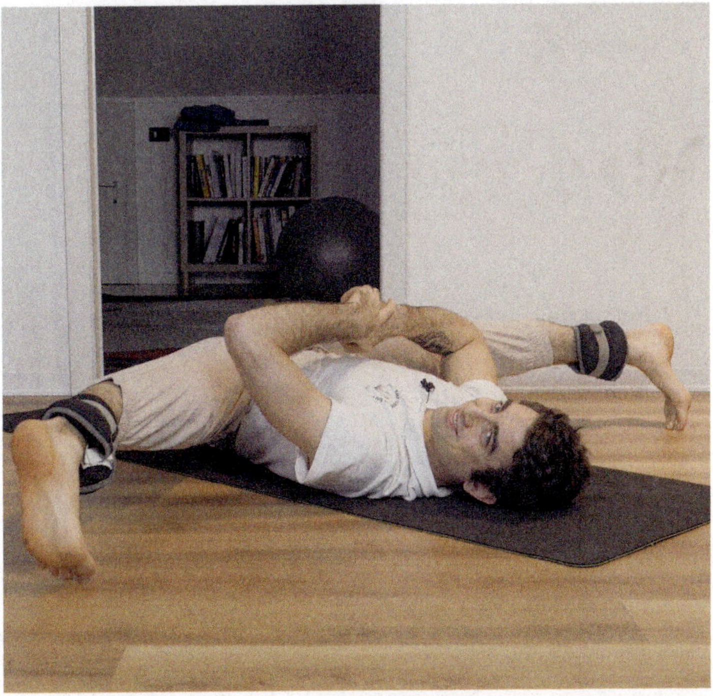

Figure 17. The Pancake Stretch.

BEGINNER WORKOUT

Sumo squat	2 sets. **First set**: Hands on the knees and push them out. 2 PNF contractions. Relaxation phases 6 breaths, PNF 10". **Second set**: hold the sumo squat as wide as you can for 30". Use a weight and let it pulls you down.
One leg squat opener	1 set per leg, 6 dynamic reps and 10 final breaths in the deepest position you can reach. Use a **weight**.
Cossack squat	2 sets, 6 reps per leg. Use some blocks under your feet if you need and spend a couple of seconds at the bottom of each rep.
Calf stretches	1 set on each leg, 3 PNF contractions. Passive phases 8 breaths, PNF 10".
Lying glutes and piriformis on floor	1 set, 3 PNF contractions. Relaxation phases 5 breaths, PNF 10".
Compass hip opener	1 set on each leg, 10 reps with a 2" pause at the bottom of each rep and a longer pause of 10 breaths on the last one.
90/90 Stretch	1 set, 20 transitions from one side to the other. Once done, perform a **pigeon pose**. 1 PNF contraction on each side. Relaxing phases 8 breaths, PNF 10".

Taylor pose	1 set, 3 PNF contractions. Relaxation phases 10 breaths, PNF 15".
Frog stretch on wall with weights	1 set, 3 PNF contractions. Relaxation phases 10 breaths, PNF 15".
Seated one leg pike	1 set, 2 PNF contractions. Relaxation phases 8 breaths, PNF 15".
Kneeling one leg pancake	1 set, 8 reps and 2 PNF contractions. Perform the reps first, then remain in the stretch and apply the PNF contractions: relaxing phases 5 breaths, PNF 10".
Chest to wall split	2 sets, 3 PNF contractions. Relaxation phases 10 breaths, PNF 15".
Seated good morning	2 sets, 6 reps. Remain in the bottom position for 2" at each rep and for 10 final seconds on the last one.
Lateral pancake on bench	1 set per side, 8 reps and 1 PNF contraction. Perform the reps **with a weight** first, then remain in the stretch and apply 1 PNF contraction. Relaxing phases 5 breaths, PNF 10".
Standing pancake stretch	2 sets, 6 dynamic repetitions where you bend and extend your legs, and 10 final breaths in the stretch, trying every 3 breaths to get a little deeper into the stretch.

ADDITIONAL NOTES

This is an example of a very good **beginner** flexibility program.

Your practice should follow your own level of flexibility: do your best to find your best stretching sensation at all times and start with the recommended poses, making sure they start to feel comfortable and progressively more accessible.

There are no particular prescriptions in terms of rest from one exercise to the other. Start an exercise when you feel fresh and well-rested, accordingly also to your time restrictions (if you have any).

Depending on your needs, you can repeat this specific workout 2 to 4 times a week. More than 4 times a week for me is not optimal for recovery, but feel free to experiment with doing something more and see how it gets eventually.

On the other days, you can train different stuff (like the splits or your upper body flexibility, using my other two books, *Splits Hacking* and *Shoulders Range*) and keep a light stretching session for the muscles involved in a pancake. Take note though that if you're training for the side split, you should combine your pancake work with your side split work, as they involved very similar groups of muscles.

Stick to your flexibility plan for at least 6/10 weeks, then measure your progress, and give the harder positions a go. If you feel good in a harder stretch, maintaining a good technique and form, then go for it and change that exercise with an easier one in your workout program. You can also feel free to experiment with plenty of other exercises you can find in the book, which are there for you to try and feel. Slowly maintain this approach until you can afford most of the positions in the intermediate program.

INTERMEDIATE WORKOUT

90/90 Stretch	1 set, 20 transitions from one side to the other. Once done, perform a **pigeon pose**. 1 PNF contraction on each side. Relaxing phases 8 breaths, PNF 10".
Sumo squat	2 sets, 10 controlled and deep reps. **Weighted.** On the last one, remain in the bottom position for 10 final seconds.
Taylor pose	1 set, 3 PNF contractions. Relaxation phases 10 breaths, PNF 15".
One leg squat opener	1 set per leg, 6 dynamic reps and 10 final breaths in the deepest position you can reach. Use a **weight**.
Cossack squat	2 sets, 6 reps per leg. Use some blocks under your feet if you need and spend a couple of seconds at the bottom of each rep.
One leg pike extension	1 set, 8 reps and 2 PNF contractions. Perform the reps first, then remain in the stretch and apply the PNF contractions: relaxing phases 5 breaths, PNF 10".
Wall hamstrings and calves	1 set per leg, 3 PNF contractions. Relaxing phases 8 breaths, PNF 10".
Frog stretch on wall with weights	1 set, 3 PNF contractions. Relaxation phases 10 breaths, PNF 15".

Lateral pancake on bench and on the floor	2 sets per side, one on the bench, one on the floor. 8 reps per side and 1 PNF contraction. Perform the reps **with a weight**, then remain in the stretch and apply 1 PNF contraction. Relaxing phases 5 breaths, PNF 10".
Standing pancake stretch	2 sets, 6 dynamic repetitions where you bend and extend your legs, and 10 final breaths in the stretch, trying every 3 breaths to get a little deeper into the stretch.
Chest to wall split	2 sets, 3 PNF contractions. Relaxation phases 10 breaths, PNF 15".
Seated good morning	2 sets, 6 reps. Remain in the bottom position for 2" at each rep and for 10 final seconds on the last one.
Butt elevated pancake, bent and straight legs	2 sets of pancake extensions with a **weight**. 8 reps per set and 10 final breaths on the last rep, where you relax with your trunk on the yoga blocks. First set with your legs bent, second set with your legs straight.
Pulling into pancake	2 sets, legs straight. 2 PNF contractions. Relaxing phases 8 breaths, PNF 10".

ADDITIONAL NOTES

This is an example of an **intermediate** flexibility program.

Your practice should follow your own level of flexibility: do your best to find your best stretching sensation at all times and start with the recommended poses, making sure they start to feel comfortable and progressively more accessible.

There are no particular prescriptions in terms of rest from one exercise to the other. Start an exercise when you feel fresh and well-rested, accordingly also to your time restrictions (if you have any).

Depending on your needs, you can repeat this specific workout 2 to 4 times a week. More than 4 times a week for me is not optimal for recovery, but feel free to experiment with doing something more and see how it gets eventually.

On the other days, you can train different stuff (like the splits or your upper body flexibility, using my other two books, *Splits Hacking* and *Shoulders Range*) and keep a light stretching session for the muscles involved in a pancake. Take note, though, that if you're training for the side split, you should combine your pancake work with your side split work, as they involved very similar groups of muscles.

Stick to your flexibility plan for at least 6/10 weeks, then measure your progress, and give the harder positions a go. If you feel good in a harder stretch, maintaining a good technique and form, then go for it and change that exercise with an easier one in your workout program. You can also feel free to experiment with plenty of other exercises you can find in the book, which are there for you to try and feel. Slowly maintain this approach until you can afford most of the positions in the advanced program.

ADVANCED WORKOUT

90/90 Stretch	1 set, 20 transitions from one side to the other. Once done, perform a **pigeon pose**. 1 PNF contraction on each side. Relaxing phases 8 breaths, PNF 10".
Sumo squat	2 sets, 10 controlled and deep reps. **Weighted.** On the last one, remain in the bottom position for 10 final seconds.
Cossack squat	2 sets, 6 reps per leg. Use some blocks under your feet if you need and spend a couple of seconds at the bottom of each rep.
Frog stretch on wall with weights	1 set, 3 PNF contractions. Relaxation phases 10 breaths, PNF 15".
Wall hamstrings and calves	1 set per leg, 3 PNF contractions. Relaxing phases 8 breaths, PNF 10".
Raising foot pancake stretch	1 set per leg, 2 PNF contractions. Relaxing phases 6 breaths, PNF 10".
Lying side split	1 set, 2 PNF contractions. Relaxing phases 8 breaths, PNF 10". Maintain a **strong** antagonist contraction for 10" after each PNF contraction.
Box split	2 set, 2 PNF contractions. Relaxing phases 8 breaths, PNF 10". Maintain a **strong** antagonist contraction for 10" after each PNF contraction.

Lateral pancake on the floor	2 sets per side, leg straight on the floor. Perform the reps **with a weight**, then remain in the stretch and apply 1 PNF contraction. Relaxing phases 5 breaths, PNF 10".
Standing pancake stretch	1 set, 6 dynamic repetitions where you bend and extend your legs, and 10 final breaths in the stretch, trying every 3 breaths to get a little deeper into the stretch.
Butt elevated straight legs pancake extension	2 sets, 8 reps. Control the repetitions and remain for 2" at the bottom of each rep. On the last one remain there with your chest on the yoga blocks or on the floor for 10 final seconds. If you're comfortable on the blocks, perform the exercise on the floor.
Pulling into pancake or pancake rolls	2 sets, 20 breaths in the position or 10 reps for the rolls. Try to stay as passive as possible, using your activations to get into the stretch.
Over-pancake	1 or 2 sets, 2 PNF contractions. Relaxing phases 6 breaths, PNF 10".
Lying pancake	1 or 2 sets, 10 to 20 breaths in the position, trying to get as deep as possible into the stretch.

ADDITIONAL NOTES

This is an example of an **advanced** flexibility program.

Your practice should follow your own level of flexibility: do your best to find your best stretching sensation at all times and start with the recommended poses, making sure they start to feel comfortable and progressively more accessible.

There are no particular prescriptions in terms of rest from one exercise to the other. Start an exercise when you feel fresh and well-rested, accordingly also to your time restrictions (if you have any).

Depending on your needs, you can repeat this specific workout 2 to 4 times a week. More than 4 times a week for me is not optimal for recovery, but feel free to experiment with doing something more and see how it gets eventually.

On the other days, you can train different stuff (like the splits or your upper body flexibility, using my other two books, *Splits Hacking* and *Shoulders Range*) and keep a light stretching session for the muscles involved in a pancake. Take note, though, that if you're training for the side split, you should combine your pancake work with your side split work, as they involved very similar groups of muscles.

This is advanced stuff. There are no fixed rules on when to make progress. Take it easy and enjoy the journey. When you feel like it, measure your progress, and give the harder positions a go. If you feel good in a harder stretch, maintaining a good technique and form, then go for it and change that exercise with an easier one in your workout program. You can also feel free to experiment with plenty of other exercises you can find in the book, which are there for you to try and feel.

Congratulations, because at this point, the pancake should be really close to mastery!

HOW TO ORGANIZE YOUR WORKOUTS

We've seen different programs so far, and I've tried to always put things in context and give you the guidelines you should follow to master your pancake and improve your lower-body flexibility. By the way, I know that organizing your flexibility workouts isn't an easy task, so I want to share with you a little secret that has helped my students and me with our flexibility training quite a lot over the past few years.

Many people ask me **what they should do if they feel sore** after a flexibility session or feel like they're "losing" their flexibility from one workout to the other. Most of the time, this is a problem of **intensity**. As you've learned in the Stretching Methodologies Chapter of this book, intensity is the amount of stretch you feel in a certain stretching position.

People who want to improve their flexibility fast go too hard too soon. They train hard every day, giving all they got each and every day. This is the perfect recipe to stress your muscles way too much and to feel sore and not well-rested as if you've "lost" some of your flexibility. What you want to do instead is to **adjust the intensity** of the stretching positions throughout the week. Let me explain this concept a little bit better. Generally speaking, you can stretch with three different levels of intensity:

- **Low intensity:** easy positions.

- **Medium intensity:** still easy positions, but slightly more uncomfortable.

- **High intensity:** uncomfortable to really uncomfortable stretching positions.

To make flexibility gains, I suggest you use the following strategy.

There are no particular limits in terms of training frequency. You can stretch **daily**, but... You want to perform a high-intensity workout **only two or three times per week**.

On the other days, you can still stretch, but with a low-intensity strategy. With a "low-intensity strategy," I mean holding the position passively without experiencing excessive discomfort. It should feel really ok and almost comfortable.

Let me show you an example right now to let you understand how to do it by yourself.

You want to train the pancake with high-intensity strategies (the ones you find in the workout templates of this book, with a weight, PNF contractions, etc.) **two times a week at max**.

On the other days, you can still stretch for the pancake, but you want to take it substantially easier. Stay in your stretching positions for a minute or two. **Little to no PNF**. **Small weights**. Not too much stretch, and that's it. Imagine covering a 10-mile distance. You can do that by running or walking. Still, they remain 10 miles. What changes is how you cover them. Here it's exactly the same: two days you run (high intensity), and two days you walk (low intensity).

Of course, you might be training more than four times a week or less, but the idea remains the same. If you feel great and well-rested with two heavy sessions per week, consider the idea of doing an additional one, reaching three heavy sessions per week, and seeing how it goes. Leave the other days light.

Another good idea may be integrating your lower-body sessions with some upper-body work. For example, let's assume you want to work on your upper-body flexibility using the bridges and/or other shoulders and upper body stretches you can find in my book: *Shoulders Range*, and work on your lower body flexibility using the splits, as you can learn in my book *Splits Hacking*. How can you arrange your weekly workouts?

Given that you may dedicate two heavy and two light sessions for each flexibility position per week, here's an idea for you, always based on four days per week.

- **Day 1**: Front Split (Heavy), Shoulders and Bridge (Heavy), Side Split and Pancake (Light).

- **Day 2**: Side Split (Heavy), Pancake (Heavy) Front Split (Light), Shoulders and Bridge (Light).

- **Day 3**: Front Split (Heavy), Shoulders and Bridge (Heavy), Side Split and Pancake (Light).

- **Day 4**: Side Split (Heavy), Pancake (Heavy) Front Split (Light), Shoulders and Bridge (Light).

In conclusion, how to structure your workouts really depends on you and on your personal needs. Unfortunately, I can't provide something that works for each person on earth. As I said at the beginning of this chapter, my purpose here is to teach you something extremely valuable: how to do it yourself. And I hope I've succeeded in that.

Remember...

—

TAKE ACTION!

TIME TO TAKE ACTION!

Now you have everything you need to achieve a flat pancake stretch. You have the exercises, the methodologies, and plenty of different training programs to play with.

What really makes a difference now is your mental attitude and consistency: people often don't realize that stretching is a practical discipline: your theoretical knowledge must serve your practice. Without practice, you (or your students) won't get nearly close to reaching your goals! So… It's time to take action now.

You can return to this book whenever you want, and I highly suggest doing so: check your form, read an exercise's explanation a few more times to make sure you got every detail of it, learn what's next, etc. The journey never really stops. You get better day by day, most of the time, without even realizing it. Try always to measure your flexibility progresses, not day by day but month by month or quarter to quarter. This way, you'll rarely be disappointed by yourself.

I hope you can use this book's exercises and programs to improve your flexibility level and reach goals you've never thought possible. Thank you for allowing me to serve you through the pages of this book. As a coach, a practitioner, and passionate about this discipline, it has truly been an honor.

What I deeply care about are the results you'll get thanks to this book. For this reason, I ask you to hit me up on any of my social media platforms, even just to say hello, and share with me how this book's exercises helped you in your flexibility journey.

Thanks,

"The Flexibility Guy" Elia Bartolini.

ACKNOWLEDGMENTS

Stretching & Flexibility. Kit Laughlin 1999, 2014.

Myofascial Pain and Dysfunction: the trigger point manual. Travell, J. G., and Simons, D. G., 1983, 1992.

DCSS, Power Mechanics For Power Lifters. Paolo Evangelista, 2011, 2014.

Fitness Posturale. Andrea Roncari, 2019.

Page P. Current concepts in muscle stretching for exercise and rehabilitation. *Int J Sports Phys Ther*. 2012;7(1):109-119.

Page, Phil. "Current concepts in muscle stretching for exercise and rehabilitation." *International journal of sports physical therapy* vol. 7,1 (2012): 109-19.

Page P. (2012). Current concepts in muscle stretching for exercise and rehabilitation. *International journal of sports physical therapy*, 7(1), 109–119.

Page P. Current concepts in muscle stretching for exercise and rehabilitation. Int J Sports Phys Ther. 2012 Feb;7(1):109-19. PMID: 22319684; PMCID: PMC3273886.

▶ YouTube

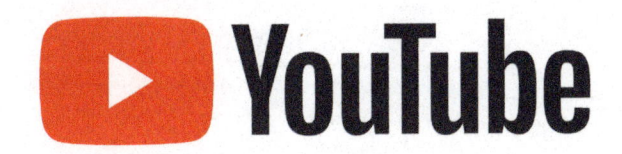

Have You Liked the Exercises That You've Learned About In This Book?

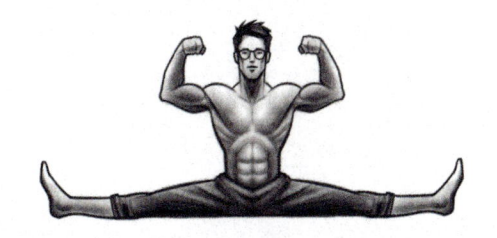

*If the Answer is Yes, Then **Subscribe** to My FREE YouTube Channel Called*
"The Flexibility Guy - Coach Elia"
Where I Share My Best Flexibility Exercises <u>Weekly</u>!

Printed in Great Britain
by Amazon